Nine Months
and a Day

A Pregnancy
and Birth Companion

Adrienne B. Lieberman
and
Linda Hughey Holt, M.D., F.A.C.O.G.

The Harvard Common Press
Boston, Massachusetts

Handy Information

First day of last menstrual period: _____

Date of conception (if known): _____

Calendar due date: _____

Ultrasound scan due date: _____

Baby's actual birthdate: _____

Mother's blood type: _____   Rh factor: _____

Father's blood type: _____   Rh factor: _____

Father's or birth partner's work phone number: _____

Mother's physician or midwife: _____

    phone number (day): _____

    phone number (night): _____

    phone number (hospital): _____

Office receptionist: _____

Nurse or caregiver's assistant: _____

    phone number: _____

Prenatal appointments (dates and times):

_____   _____   _____

_____   _____   _____

_____   _____   _____

_____   _____   _____

_____   _____   _____

Childbirth class instructor: _____

    phone number: _____

Prenatal classes (dates and times):

_____   _____

_____   _____

_____   _____

_____   _____

Babycare, breastfeeding, or other classes (class, date, and time):

_____

_____

_____

Doula: _____

     phone number: _____

La Leche League leader: _____

     phone number: _____

Lactation consultant: _____

     phone number: _____

Pharmacy: _____

     phone number: _____

Health plan: _____

     phone number: _____

     Mother's ID number: _____

Baby's doctor: _____

     phone number (day): _____

     phone number (night): _____

     phone number (hospital): _____

     office receptionist: _____

Newborn checkup (date and time): _____

Postpartum checkup (date and time): _____

The Harvard Common Press
535 Albany Street
Boston, Massachusetts 02118

www.harvardcommonpress.com

Printed in the United States of America
Printed on acid-free paper

The ISBN for *Nine Months and A Day* is now 1-55832-318-X.
It was originally published with ISBN 1-55832-150-0.

The Library of Congress has cataloged the earlier printing as follows:

Lieberman, Adrienne B.

   Nine months and a day : a pregnancy, labor, and delivery companion
/ Adrienne B. Lieberman and Linda Hughey Holt.
     p.   cm.
   Includes bibliographical references and index.
   ISBN 1-55832-150-0 (pbk. : alk. paper)
   1. Pregnancy. 2. Childbirth. 3. Infants—Care. I. Holt,
Linda Hughey. II. Title.
RG525.H56 2000
618.2—dc21   99-025178

Special bulk-order discounts are available on this and other Harvard Common Press books. Companies and organizations may purchase books for premiums or for resale, or may arrange a custom edition, by contacting the Marketing Director at the address above.

Cover design by Night & Day Design
Text design by Eclipse Publishing Services
Woodcut illustrations by Ruth J. Flanigan; all others by Ruth Linstromberg

10 9 8 7 6 5 4 3 2 1

Contents

Acknowledgments

Thanks to Harvard Common Press for inviting us to do this book and to the talented people who nurtured it through a long gestation to its eventual arrival. Special thanks to Debra Hudak for patient oversight, Linda Ziedrich for meticulous editing, Mark Corsey for a lively design, Ruth Linstromberg for her instructive illustrations, and Ruth J. Flanigan for the delightful woodcuts. Our clients over many years have made it a joy to labor in the field of pregnancy and birth. And our families have kept our home lives full and fun while we worked. With great expectations, we happily dedicate this book to a new generation of parents and babies.

Introduction

If you're pregnant or expecting to be expecting, congratulations! A life-changing adventure awaits you, beginning with the months of pregnancy and your baby's birthday. This book aims to guide you through these exciting first steps. The explanations and suggestions offered here, along with the marginal notes you add, will inform your ongoing conversation with your prenatal caregiver. Your close working partnership with this person can help you arrive at your shared goal: the safe and satisfying beginning of a brand-new life.

You may opt to see a physician or a midwife for your prenatal care. To avoid the tiresome repetition of *your doctor or midwife,* we'll call this medical professional *your caregiver* or *your birth attendant.* And, because babies come in two equally delicious flavors, we've tried to divide pronoun references fairly between *him* and *her.*

Using This Book

We hope you'll find all of the information in this book helpful. The features described below may be particularly useful in certain situations.

 Advice and Instructions Lists: These checklists, identified by the pencil and paper icon, provide step-by-step instructions to help you carry out or prepare for particular tasks, such as exercising safely or breastfeeding.

 Question Lists: These lists, identified by the notepad icon, will help you remember which questions to ask when evaluating candidates for such important roles as birth attendant or childbirth class instructor.

 Partner Support: Your birth partner may find especially helpful these text sections, identified by the holding hands icon. The text sometimes provides specific, hands-on advice, such as "enjoy watching and feeling your baby's movements together". Other times, reviewing the material discussed near an icon will increase your partner's awareness of your need for emotional support.

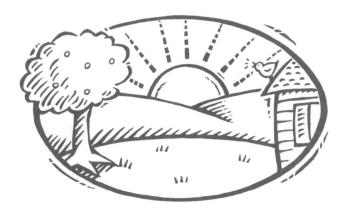

CHAPTER 1

First Things First

Because the most important stages of your baby's development may happen before you even discover you're pregnant, you can give your baby the best possible start by planning your pregnancy. Already pregnant, or think you might be? Skim this section, or skip ahead to "Pregnant? How to Tell" (page 5).

---❤---

Planning Ahead

If you're considering getting pregnant in the near future, it's ideal to do these things first:

1. Schedule a preconception exam. This checkup involves a complete physical examination, a discussion of your medical history and current health habits, laboratory tests, and any necessary shots. Plenty of time should also be included for your questions.

2. Consider genetic counseling. Your ethnic background, family history, or age—or your partner's—may put you at a higher-

than-average risk of bearing a child with a genetic defect. A genetic counselor can tell you what risks you face, describe the available screening tests, acquaint you with the benefits and limitations of testing, explain the choices you may need to make when you learn the results, and offer support to help you make these choices. Before pregnancy, you and your partner can undergo blood screening for any one of several diseases that can strike one out of four pregnancies in women who share a defective gene with their partners. You may also choose to undergo genetic screening if you have suffered two or more unexplained miscarriages; have previously delivered a baby with a chromosomal problem; have a close relative with a genetic disease such as hemophilia, cystic fibrosis, or muscular dystrophy; or have been exposed to radiation or dangerous chemicals.

3. Address health problems. Medical improvements allow women with a variety of health problems to undertake pregnancy confidently and to anticipate healthy births (see Chapter 6). But if you have a medical condition such as diabetes or high blood pressure, it's best to avoid getting pregnant until you have discussed your plans with your physician and a prenatal caregiver. Doing so allows your medical team to check the safety of your medications and plan for the best possible management of your pregnancy.

    Be sure to ask about any medication you take, no matter how harmless it seems. Some of the medications regularly prescribed for acne, arthritis, epilepsy, heart disease, lupus, and psychiatric disorders can harm a growing baby. Likewise, ingredients in many popular over-the-counter drugs could pose a potential threat to your baby. Find a safer alternative before you get pregnant.

4. Get tested. Blood tests can reveal whether you're immune to certain diseases and whether you need treatment or vaccination for others. You may be tested for—

    ▲ hypothyroidism
    ▲ rubella (German measles)
    ▲ chicken pox
    ▲ hepatitis B
    ▲ toxoplasmosis

▲ tuberculosis

▲ cytomegalovirus

▲ human immunodeficiency virus (HIV)

▲ other sexually transmitted diseases, such as chlamydia, syphilis, and gonorrhea

A recent study indicates that children born to mothers with untreated hypothyroidism later scored lower on IQ tests than did children of healthy or treated mothers.

If tests indicate that you lack immunity to rubella or chicken pox—childhood diseases that can threaten your baby if you catch them during pregnancy—you can be inoculated against these illnesses. But you'll need to put off getting pregnant for three months following either vaccination.

Vaccination before or even during pregnancy is recommended for hepatitis B, a serious liver disease.

Unknowing carriers of HIV can pass this infection to their babies. Once a carrier is identified, however, she can be treated. Treatment for HIV cuts a baby's risk of infection and boosts his mother's life expectancy.

5. See your dentist. It's best to avoid routine X-rays and minimize anesthesia and pain medications while pregnant. In addition, untreated gum disease can trigger labor prematurely. So schedule a dental exam, get your teeth cleaned, and have any necessary work done beforehand, if possible.

6. Get into shape. A normal weight protects you during pregnancy and birth. If you start pregnancy well over a healthy weight, you risk complications that include high blood pressure, preeclampsia, gestational diabetes, a too-big baby, and a cesarean or operative delivery. If you are serviously underweight, you may have trouble getting or staying pregnant, and you face an increased risk of having a baby born prematurely or at low birth weight. Avoid fad diets; they risk your and your baby's health. Instead, ask your doctor to refer you to a nutritionist. Also, consider beginning a regular exercise routine.

7. Kick harmful habits. The most common preventable danger to an unborn baby is his mother's use of alcohol, tobacco, and nonmedical drugs such as cocaine (see pages 54 to 57). Don't be afraid to speak up if you need help quitting any of these dangerous habits; see "Resources" for referrals.

8. Steer clear of dangers. Your work or hobbies could pose a threat to your unborn baby if you are regularly exposed to illness, X-rays, or chemicals. You may need to observe certain precautions, take a leave of absence, or even switch jobs. For example, if your children are in school or daycare, or if you work with young children, you may be exposed to common childhood illnesses such as chicken pox or fifth disease, either of which could cause serious fetal problems if you lack immunity. If your house is being renovated or if you work as a house painter, consider having your blood tested for lead. Serious problems, including miscarriage, fetal abnormalities, and premature birth, have also been linked to these agents:

   ▲ anesthetic gases, such as nitrous oxide
   ▲ cadmium, used in batteries, electroplating, and pigments for paints, inks, and plastics
   ▲ carbon monoxide, present in exhaust gases
   ▲ cytotoxic drugs, such as methotrexate, which is used in treating cancer and other diseases
   ▲ ethylene oxide, used in making antifreeze as well as detergents
   ▲ halogenated hydrocarbons, such as PBBs, PCBs, vinyl chloride, and tetrachloroethylene, used in dry cleaning solvents, foam-blowing agents, fire extinguishers, fumigants, refrigerants, and aerosol propellants
   ▲ hexachlorophene, used in antiseptic cleaning agents
   ▲ mercury, used in thermometers, paints, pesticides, and dental fillings (mercury amalgam fillings pose no risk, but dental workers may be exposed to mercury vapors)
   ▲ organic solvents found in paints, pesticides, adhesives, lacquers, and cleaning agents

For other dangers to avoid during pregnancy, see pages 54 and 75.

How about video display terminals (VDTs)? Years ago, reports suggested that VDTs may have caused miscarriages and birth defects in pregnant women who worked in front of computers. VDTs do produce X-rays, but their radiation stays within the terminals. In 1997 the National Institute for Occupational Safety and Health reported that women who work at VDTs all day have no more risk of having a premature or low-birthweight baby than women with similar jobs who do not use VDTs.

Is it safe to use your microwave oven during pregnancy? Yes, if the door seals properly. For insurance, though, avoid standing in front of the oven while it's operating.

9. Eat well, and focus on folic acid. A nutritious diet boosts your chances to get pregnant and prepares your body to nourish your baby. In particular, a high intake of the B vitamin folic acid, or folacin, before pregnancy and during the early months helps prevent neural tube defects. These defects include spina bifida, "open spine," which can cause paralysis from the waist down. Folic acid may also help prevent cleft palate and cleft lip.

   Folic acid is naturally present in fresh fruits and vegetables, dried beans and peas, and whole grains. In addition, refined flour, breads and pasta made with refined flour, and breakfast cereals now come fortified with this crucial nutrient. But during pregnancy a woman's need for folic acid doubles. So ask your caregiver about taking a prenatal multivitamin supplement containing this important vitamin. The recommended dietary allowance (RDA) of folic acid for pregnant women is 400 micrograms (.4 milligrams), but many experts believe pregnant women should get 800 micrograms (.8 milligrams) a day from conception, and most prenatal multivitamin supplements contain this amount.

   You can't overdose on folic acid from food, but experts recommend against taking more than 1,000 micrograms (1 milligram) of supplemental folic acid per day unless you face a high risk for giving birth to a baby with a neural tube defect. If so, your caregiver will probably prescribe a much higher dose of folic acid—4 milligrams a day—beginning a month before pregnancy and continuing through the first trimester.

10. Check your health coverage (see page 6).

—— ♥ ——

Pregnant? How to Tell

Some women know exactly when they conceived, while others don't even suspect they're pregnant for the first month or two. Missing a period seems an obvious sign, but some women experience implantation bleeding—slight spotting—as the embryo nestles into the uterus, and they confuse this with an actual period. These are other common symptoms of early pregnancy:

▲ intense fatigue
▲ nausea or vomiting
▲ bloating or cramping
▲ breast tenderness
▲ frequent urination

You can confirm your suspicions by taking an over-the-counter pregnancy test, available at the drugstore for about fifteen or twenty dollars. Like the tests given in doctor's offices, home pregnancy tests recognize human chorionic gonadotropin (hCG). This hormone, produced by the developing placenta, is detectable in the mother's blood and urine within a week or two after conception. If you follow the instructions to the letter, home tests are about 99 percent accurate. But health problems such as a thyroid disorder, and medications including aspirin, can cause you to test pregnant when you're not. Less often, testing too early or an ectopic pregnancy (see page 21) can make a test come out negative even though you are pregnant. So you may want to check your first result with a second test a day or two later.

Positive test results should spur you to avoid dangers (see pages 4, 54, and 75), eat well (see page 44), and get your first prenatal checkup. As early in pregnancy as possible, you'll need to decide where to give birth and who should be your birth attendant. It's also a good idea to look at your health coverage.

— ♥ —
Checking Your Health Plan and Work Leave

Read over your policy or ask your insurance representative exactly what it covers, what it excludes, whether you'll be responsible for deductibles or copayments, and how to enroll your newborn.

Maternity benefits vary from policy to policy. While some policies cover just about everything—prenatal tests, hospital stay, and intensive care if your baby needs it—others pay only a percentage of standard obstetric costs and exclude pediatric fees. You may want to supplement a limited policy with major medical insurance to spare yourself the huge costs of a serious pediatric

Unplanned Pregnancy: Do Contraceptive Pills or Implants, Spermicides, or IUDs Pose a Risk?

Birth control doesn't always work. If you conceived while taking birth control pills or after getting a Norplant insert or Depo-Provera injection, you may be worried about how the hormones in these contraceptives may affect your developing baby. Discuss these concerns with your caregiver. You'll probably be reassured that your baby faces minimal risk from exposure to contraceptive hormones. Likewise, experts say, the spermicides used in vaginal creams and condom lubricants pose no threat to babies conceived during the use of these products.

Pregnancy with an IUD in place does raise your risk of miscarriage, ectopic pregnancy (see page 21), and serious infection. If you experience a late or unusual period with an IUD in place, take an early pregnancy test. If it's positive, contact your caregiver immediately. You'll be given an ultrasound examination to identify the location of the embryo as well as of the IUD. An ectopic pregnancy must be terminated with medication or surgery. If the embryo is in your uterus and the IUD string is accessible, your caregiver should remove the device to reduce your risk of infection. An inaccessible IUD will usually be delivered along with the placenta.

illness or extended hospitalization. Here's a basic insurance checklist:

▲ Study your company's maternity and newborn coverage. Pay attention to exclusions for pre-existing conditions and complications before and after birth, lists of approved physicians and midwives, required preauthorizations for certain treatments, and sign-up procedures for newborns.

▲ If you and your partner are insured through both your employers, make sure you understand "primary" and "secondary" coverage qualifications.

▲ Anticipate any changes you may need to make in your medical coverage if you plan to take an extended leave from work after the baby comes.

▲ Consider life or disability insurance to safeguard your family should you or your partner die or become disabled.

In addition, check your employer's parental leave policies. Will you get paid time off? If so, how much? Find out whether you'll be able to apply vacation time, sick days, or short-term disability leave to extend or pay for your planned maternity leave. The 1993 Family and Medical Leave Act requires employers with more than 50 employees to offer women and men 12 weeks of unpaid leave for a birth or adoption. The Pregnancy Discrimination Act obliges employers with more than 15 workers to provide the same leave and job security to pregnant women as to disabled employees. Several states also mandate paid maternity benefits. Call your state department of labor to see whether your state is one that treats maternity leave the same as disability leave.

Birth Place and Delivery Attendants

Where you give birth and who attends the birth are closely connected. If you have a particular hospital or birthing center in mind, the policies at that institution will state which medical professionals may attend your delivery. On the other hand, if you choose a specific caregiver to deliver your baby, she or he may be licensed to deliver babies in some settings but not others. The following sections describe some of the issues to consider in selecting a birth place and delivery attendants.

Selecting a Birth Place

Where you give birth may be limited by your health plan or where you live. If possible, choose a birth place within a half hour's drive from your home. The one you select helps determine who attends your birth—your doctor or midwife. A caregiver may be able to deliver babies at several different hospitals, or only at one. Some caregivers attend births in birthing centers or in private homes.

HOSPITAL BIRTH   In the United States, most babies—99 out of 100 at last count—begin life in a hospital. If you have a choice of hospitals, you can find the best one by getting recommendations from friends who have recently given birth or from local childbirth educators. If possible, tour the hospitals before making your final selection.

Hospital Birth During the tour, you may want to ask some of these questions:

Does the hospital offer classes on childbirth, breastfeeding, and infant care, including CPR (cardiopulmonary resuscitation)?

What does an average stay cost?

How long is an average stay? In most but not all hospitals, maternity stays currently average about two days for a vaginal birth and four days for a cesarean.

What type of nursing care is offered laboring women and new mothers?

Will I be able to labor, deliver, and recover in the same room? LDR (labor-delivery-recovery) rooms represent a big improvement over the separate labor, delivery, and recovery rooms of a generation ago. Some hospitals have gone a step further and put in LDRP (labor-delivery-recovery-postpartum) rooms.

What helpful tools do you offer for comfort in labor? These may include furniture and devices that provide support in various positions, such as birthing beds, birthing balls, and birthing stools, and devices to soothe laboring women with water, such as showers, deep bathtubs, and, less frequently, birthing tubs.

How many people will be able to stay with me during the birth? Most hospitals permit one labor partner; some hospitals welcome extra supporters (see "Doulas," page 151); and some hospitals even extend the welcome to the baby's siblings, if they have taken a class (see page 152).

Question list continues on page 10

Hospital Birth During the tour, you may want to ask some of these questions:

Question list continued from page 9

Will I be permitted to eat and drink during labor? Some hospitals allow laboring women to drink clear fluids, while others permit only ice chips. Prohibiting solid food and unclear liquids, a standard precaution when general anesthesia is anticipated, may be unnecessary during labor.

Are some procedures—for example, electronic fetal monitoring or intravenous lines (IVs, see page 137)—routine?

Will I be encouraged to move around during labor and experiment with different positions, such as squatting, for birth? Are the beds equipped with squatting bars for support in this position?

What percentage of the women who deliver in the hospital receive Pitocin (see page 138)?

What percentage receive epidural anesthesia (see page 150)?

What percentage end up with cesareans (see page 142)?

Will my partner(s) be allowed in the room if I need a cesarean?

Are emergency obstetric services, such as anesthesia, available in the hospital at any hour?

In what cases are sick newborns transferred to another hospital? Where do they go?

Can my baby stay with me around the clock after the birth? What rooming-in options do you offer (see page 195)?

Can my partner stay overnight after the birth? Some hospitals provide double beds or cots for partners; others let them sleep in a chair or recliner, but many require them to go home.

What are postpartum visiting hours? Can healthy siblings visit?

Do you provide a home visit by a nurse after the birth?

OUT-OF-HOSPITAL BIRTH   Only 1 percent of babies are born out of the hospital in the United States. Two out of three of these babies greet the world at home, while about one out of three is born in a freestanding birth center. Some women feel comfortable and safe giving birth in these settings, where they can avoid routine interventions such as electronic fetal monitoring and intravenous (IV) lines. However, technological aids such as epidural anesthesia are unavailable in out-of-hospital settings.

Birthing-center Delivery If you're considering a birthing-center delivery, you may want to ask some of these questions on a tour:

Are you licensed by the state or accredited by the Commission for the Accreditation of Birth Centers? Licensing or accreditation indicates high safety standards.

Who will be my birth attendant? Most birthing centers are run by certified nurse-midwives (see page 13), who contract with physicians for backup care. Others are operated by obstetricians or family practitioners, with nurse-midwives as staff members.

What is the total cost of birth, and what services are included (childbirth classes, prenatal care, postpartum care, postpartum home visit)?

Do you provide birthing balls, birthing stools, or birthing beds?

Are birthing rooms equipped with showers, deep bathtubs, or birthing tubs? Can I stay in the tub for both labor and birth?

How close is the nearest hospital?

What percentage of women require transfer to the hospital during labor or after the birth? What are the most common reasons for transfer?

Will the doctor or midwife from the birthing center continue to provide care for me if I must be transferred?

If the baby requires immediate pediatric care, who will provide it?

Only healthy women at no special risk for complications should consider out-of-hospital birth, which may be attended by a physician or a midwife. Careful screening during pregnancy will identify women who should give birth in the hospital—those who have high blood pressure, anemia, or premature contractions, for example.

Even with careful screening, as many as one quarter of the women who plan out-of-hospital births get transferred to the hospital during labor. If you're considering an out-of-hospital birth, consider the possibility that you may need to change your plans.

As a compromise between hospital and home, a small minority of women choose to have their babies in freestanding birthing centers. These centers must provide quick access to a nearby hospital that offers complete obstetric and neonatal care. Fees at birthing centers, covered by most insurance companies, average 50 percent less than standard hospital fees.

If you think there's no place like home for birth—and most women who choose out-of-hospital birth share this view—you should live reasonably close to a hospital where your birth attendant has backup arrangements. Your home-birth caregiver needs a smooth transfer system to avoid confusion and delay in the event of an emergency. Although nonemergency situations such as lengthy labor cause most home-to-hospital transfers, emergencies sometimes happen. Ask your caregiver what will happen if you need to be transferred quickly. During pregnancy, make plans to meet the physician who will provide emergency hospital care if you need it.

Although not all health plans cover home birth, the costs tend to be low and parental satisfaction high.

Who Attends Deliveries?

In the United States, physicians currently attend about 92 out of 100 births; midwives take care of the other 8 percent. Most of the doctors who attend births are **obstetrician-gynecologists (OB/GYNs).** Their surgical training qualifies them to care for obstetric and gynecological problems and to perform cesareans.

After passing special oral and written exams, an OB/GYN can become board-certified. Many competent physicians, however, are not board-certified. These include doctors who trained very recently and have not yet passed the exam as well as doctors who trained years ago, before board certification became common. But board certification shows that a physician has made a successful effort to maintain professional standards.

Some OB/GYNs complete a fellowship that qualifies them to manage high-risk pregnancy and birth. These subspecialists— **perinatologists**—practice only in major medical centers, where they manage the problem pregnancies that require their special skills. After passing an additional oral and written exam, perinatologists can become board-certified for their subspecialty.

A minority of birth attendants are **family practitioners.** They care for normal pregnancies and consider the health-care needs of the entire family. You may appreciate the convenience of having one person serve as doctor for both you and your baby. If you choose a family practitioner, ask which specialist this doctor will call if complications arise during your pregnancy.

An increasing number of pregnant women seek midwifery care because it emphasizes the normality of pregnancy and birth. Midwives usually schedule longer prenatal appointments, accompany a woman through her entire labor and delivery, and offer instruction in baby care. About 95 of 100 midwife-assisted births are attended by **certified nurse-midwives (CNMs),** registered nurses who have completed one or more years of special training in midwifery. These professionals, who specialize in the care of healthy women and their newborns, always practice with the backup of obstetrician-gynecologists. Almost all deliveries attended by CNMs take place in hospitals and freestanding birth centers, though some take place in private homes.

Independent midwives are sometimes called lay midwives, direct-entry midwives (because they entered the profession directly, not through nursing), or empiric midwives. These practitioners may or may not be certified or licensed. Licensed midwives, who typically attend birth only in out-of-hospital settings, have met qualifications that vary from state to state. But not all states license independent midwives. Unlicensed midwives, with varying levels of training and skill, also attend home births.

MAKING THE CHOICE   Choosing the right caregiver depends partly on your prospects at the start of pregnancy. If you have diabetes

> **Choosing the Right Caregiver** Call several caregivers' offices. On the phone, you might ask:
>
> *What are the birth attendant's training and qualifications?*
>
> *Where does the doctor or midwife attend births?*
>
> *What does prenatal care, birth, and postpartum care cost? What is included in the fee? When must the fee be paid? What part of the fee is covered by my health plan?*
>
> *Does the birth attendant charge for an initial interview?*
>
> *How long is a typical prenatal appointment? Can I request extra time if I have a lot of questions?*

or another serious medical condition, or if your pregnancy develops complications, you'll most likely see an obstetrician and perhaps consult with a perinatologist. If you're healthy and your pregnancy progresses normally, your range of options may include obstetricians, family practitioners, and midwives.

If you have a choice of caregivers, get referrals from satisfied friends with babies, a labor and delivery nurse, or a childbirth educator. Phone calls to several caregivers' offices can provide you with some basic information.

The information you get during these phone interviews should help you narrow your list to two or three likely candidates. Bring your partner along for interview sessions with the birth attendants you're considering. Listen to how each caregiver responds to your questions, and note red flags such as annoyance with your questions or a dismissal of your concerns. The specific answers to these questions may be less important than your potential caregiver's problem-solving approach and attitude toward working with you.

If after starting prenatal care you have doubts about your choice, express them, and then listen to what your caregiver has to say. If you and your caregiver can't reach a meeting of minds, it's much better to switch to another practitioner than to persist in an unhappy partnership.

Questions for Caregivers Compile a list of questions about the issues you care most about. You may wish to ask:

How can I reach you in case of an emergency?

What advice do you offer about nutrition, working, travel, and exercise?

What type of childbirth classes do you recommend?

For what percentage of your clients do you actually attend births? If you're not there for my delivery, who will cover for you? Can I meet this person? Will your substitute honor the agreements we make about labor and delivery?

How much time do you typically spend with a woman in labor?

How do you encourage your clients to cope with labor pain (see page 147)?

What helpers can accompany me to labor and birth?

Do you have routine orders for patients in labor? What are they?

Can they be adapted for my preferences?

How do you advise women who prefer to avoid episiotomies (see page 139)?

What proportion of your clients have cesareans? What are the commonest reasons for performing surgery? How can I reduce my risk of needing a cesarean?

A Family Affair

Family ties shift during pregnancy. With your first pregnancy, you and your partner will form a new relationship as parents. Your own parents may also need time to adjust to being pushed up the generational ladder. With subsequent pregnancies, your older children will struggle to accommodate themselves to the newest addition. Classes on parenting, grandparenting, and being a sibling can help ease these challenging transitions.

Your relationship with your partner will probably undergo the biggest change during your first pregnancy. Becoming a parent is both exhilarating and terrifying. Along with all the excitement, many partners find themselves overwhelmed with the many responsibilities new parenthood entails. Your own partner may also feel—

▲ very protective of you and the baby;
▲ left out, as you become increasingly absorbed in your pregnancy;
▲ uncomprehending of the fact that he'll soon be a father;
▲ worried about how he will react during the birth and afterward; or
▲ uncomfortable right along with you (see "couvade," page 27).

To strengthen your bond during pregnancy, try doing these things together: Listen to each other's complaints, fears, and hopes. Fantasize about how your life will be after the baby comes, and tell each other what qualities will make you great parents. Stay physically intimate: Enjoy watching and feeling your baby's movements together, massage each other with oil, and be flexible and inventive about sex (see page 73). As a pair, attend prenatal appointments, choose a doctor for your baby, take childbirth classes, choose your baby's name, and decorate and equip the nursery. A few weeks before the birth, prepare some meals together that you can store in the freezer. And do some things you'll need to postpone for a while after the baby comes: Splurge on a weekend at a hotel, go out for a fancy dinner, sleep late, and enjoy a leisurely breakfast in bed.

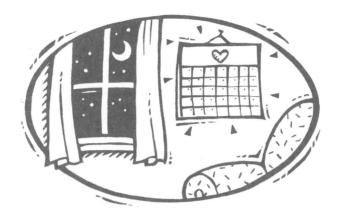

CHAPTER 2

Your Pregnancy, Month by Month

As the months go by, your baby develops, your body changes, and your mind expands to include the idea of your growing passenger. Little by little, you begin to feel more like a parent to your baby. Use these pages to remind yourself of the important things you need to do. In the margins, you and your partner can note milestones, such as the big day you each first felt your baby move.

A Monthly Guide

First Trimester

MONTH 1
Your baby grows:

- ▲ Fertilization happens about two weeks after your last menstrual period.
- ▲ By the end of the first month of pregnancy, the two-week-old embryo has nestled into the uterus, where the placenta, amniotic sac, and amniotic fluid begin to form.
- ▲ Less than one-fourth of an inch long, the embryo is about as big as a grain of rice.

Your body changes:

- ▲ You miss your period.
- ▲ You need to urinate more often.
- ▲ Your breasts may feel full and heavy; your nipples may become sensitive.
- ▲ Your lower abdomen may feel bloated or achy.
- ▲ You may feel fatigued.
- ▲ You may begin to feel nauseated, and you may vomit.

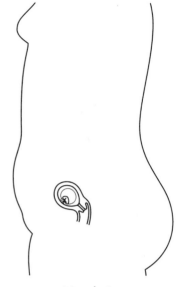

Month 1

Things to do:

- ▲ Take a pregnancy test to confirm your pregnancy.
- ▲ Sign up for prenatal care (see pages 8 to 15, and Chapter 3).
- ▲ If you smoke, drink, or use nonmedical drugs, quit immediately (see pages 54 to 57).
- ▲ Stop taking any unnecessary medication; if in doubt, ask your caregiver.
- ▲ Consult your caregiver about taking a multivitamin containing folic acid (see page 5). Unless medically advised otherwise, avoid consuming more than 1,000 micrograms (1 milligram) per day in a supplement.
- ▲ Eat well, according to your appetite.

MONTH 2
Your baby grows:

- ▲ The circulatory system develops; the heart beats by 25 days after conception.
- ▲ The brain and spinal column form; the large head has eyes, ears, and the beginnings of a mouth.
- ▲ Arm buds appear 26 days after conception, and leg buds appear by 28 days.

▲ The kidneys, the liver, the digestive tract, and a primitive umbilical cord begin to form.

▲ Now about an inch long, the embryo weighs about one-third of an ounce.

Your body changes:

▲ Your blood volume begins to expand.

▲ You may experience fatigue, nausea, constipation, heartburn, gas, food aversions or cravings, or headaches (see Chapter 5).

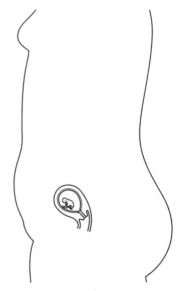

Month 2

Things to do:

▲ Consider keeping a pregnancy journal or asking your partner to take a picture of you each month to document your body's changes.

▲ Discuss the pros and cons of chorionic villus sampling (CVS), page 38, and first-trimester Down syndrome screening, page 36.

▲ Consider taking an early-bird childbirth class or a prenatal exercise class.

▲ If you're nauseated, eat frequent, small meals of bland but wholesome foods; if you're tired, too, have your partner take over most of the cooking and shopping.

MONTH 3
Your baby grows:

▲ By the eighth week after conception, bone cells replace softer cartilage cells in the skeleton, and the embryo becomes a fetus.

▲ Features begin to develop on the face—eyelids, a nose, ears, lips, and a tongue. Tooth buds develop, too.

▲ The arms have hands with fingers, soft nail beds, and fingerprints; the legs have knees, ankles, and toes.

- ▲ Tiny arms and legs begin to move.
- ▲ The fetus can smile, frown, suck her thumb, swallow amniotic fluid, and urinate in it (the amniotic fluid is completely replaced about every three hours).
- ▲ The fetal heartbeat can be heard with an ultrasound stethoscope, called a Doppler.
- ▲ The fetus is now about 3 inches long and weighs about 1 ounce.

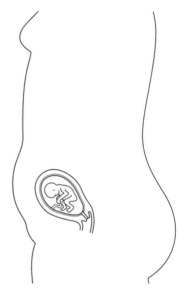

Month 3

Your body changes:

- ▲ During this trimester, you will probably gain about five pounds, though some mothers lose weight.
- ▲ You begin to feel and look more pregnant.

Things to do:

- ▲ Let out some waistlines or choose clothes with elastic waistbands.
- ▲ Scout out good sources for maternity clothes; you'll probably need them next month.
- ▲ Discuss the pros and cons of amniocentesis (see page 39).

Miscarriage and Ectopic Pregnancy

At least one in five diagnosed pregnancies ends in **miscarriage,** the loss of an embryo or fetus before the twentieth week of pregnancy. Many miscarriages result from genetic abnormalities. Maternal infection, exposure to toxic substances, abnormalities in the uterus or cervix, and serious injury can also be to blame. Normal activities, such as bending, moderate exercise, sex, or even a glass of beer or wine, do *not* cause miscarriage. Most women who miscarry will eventually be able to have a healthy baby.

Several symptoms indicate that a miscarriage is possible or inevitable, or that it has already happened. Though bleeding and pain can pass without a problem, call your caregiver immediately if you experience—

- ▲ vaginal bleeding,
- ▲ abdominal pain, or
- ▲ cramping.

About 2 percent of pregnancies begin to grow outside the uterus, dooming the fetus and putting the mother's life at risk. **Ectopic pregnancy,** which almost always occurs in one of the fallopian tubes, typically requires emergency surgery. With early diagnosis, though, an ectopic pregnancy may sometimes be treated with methotrexate. This cancer medication dissolves the rapidly growing embryonic tissue before it ruptures the tube. Saving the tube boosts the odds for a successful next pregnancy.

Unfortunately, it can be hard to diagnose an ectopic pregnancy early, because an expectant mother may notice no symptoms until her tube has ruptured. Or she may experience only subtle symptoms— light vaginal bleeding and abdominal pain—about four to six weeks after her first missed period when a life-threatening **tubal rupture** is imminent.

When a fallopian tube ruptures, symptoms may include—

- ▲ constant, severe abdominal pain that sometimes radiates to the shoulders,
- ▲ heavy bleeding, and
- ▲ chills and fainting (from blood loss).

Ectopic pregnancies have been on the rise lately because more women have pelvic inflammatory disease (PID) from chlamydia and other sexually transmitted diseases. PID scars the tubes, blocking the passage of the fertilized egg to the uterus. Though the cause of ectopic pregnancy often remains a mystery, other risk factors include—

- ▲ conditions that could damage the tubes, such as a ruptured appendix, a ruptured ovarian cyst, tubal surgery, or a previous ectopic pregnancy;
- ▲ the use of an intrauterine birth control device (IUD); and
- ▲ being the daughter of a woman who took DES during pregnancy (see page 104).

Second Trimester

MONTH 4

Your baby grows:

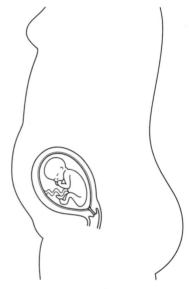

Month 4

- ▲ The umbilical cord and fetal organs are all formed; from now on, the fetus mostly just grows bigger.
- ▲ The external sex organs become visibly male or female.
- ▲ Fingernails and toenails begin to form.
- ▲ Downy hair called lanugo covers the fetus's thin, transparent skin.
- ▲ The fetus sleeps, wakes, and hears; he also rolls around in the amniotic fluid.
- ▲ The fetus is now about 5 to 6 inches long and weighs about a quarter of a pound.

Your body changes:

- ▲ This month, your abdomen begins to swell.
- ▲ If you are very thin or have had a baby before, you may feel fetal movements about 16 weeks after your last menstrual period.

Things to do:

- ▲ Establish or resume an exercise routine if you feel up to it; regular, moderate exercise is healthy for you and your baby (see Chapter 4).
- ▲ Consider notifying people at work—your boss first— about your pregnancy if you don't want them to guess.

MONTH 5

Your baby grows:

- ▲ The fetus sucks her thumb and may get the hiccups.

▲ Hair, eyelashes, and eye-brows begin to grow.
▲ The heartbeat can be heard with an ordinary stethoscope.
▲ The fetus is 8 to 12 inches long and weighs about a pound.

Your body changes:

▲ By mid-pregnancy, your milk glands contain co-lostrum, or pre-milk.
▲ If you haven't felt fetal movement before, you begin to feel it now.

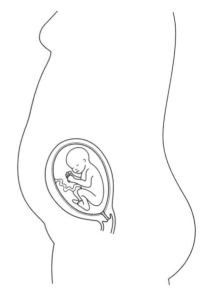

Month 5

Things to do:

▲ Sign up for childbirth classes (see page 123).
▲ Explore your employer's prenatal leave policy (see page 8). Begin to prepare your children for their new sibling by pointing out other families with new babies, reading books about birth and babies, and reviewing your children's own baby pictures. Plan to enroll them in hospital sibling classes and to complete any necessary bed or bedroom switches well before the baby arrives.

MONTH 6
Your baby grows:

▲ A cheesy protective coating called vernix covers the fetus's red, wrinkled skin.
▲ The fetal eyes open.
▲ Meconium (fetal stool) begins to fill the fetal bowel.
▲ The fetal lungs remain undeveloped; if born now, a baby might survive, but only with very specialized care.
▲ The fetus is about 11 to 14 inches long and weighs between 1 and 1½ pounds.

Your body changes:

▲ Weight gain typically peaks during this month.

▲ You feel vigorous fetal movement.

▲ Symptoms of late pregnancy—such as heartburn, backache, varicose veins, hemorrhoids, and abdominal pain from the stretching of the round ligaments (see Chapter 5)—may begin to demand your attention.

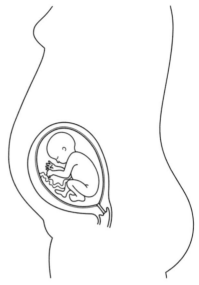

Month 6

Things to do:

▲ Prepare for parenthood: read books and articles, talk to experienced parents, and sign up for classes on baby care and breastfeeding.

▲ If you plan to breastfeed, see whether your nipples stick out when you gently compress your areola (the colored area around the nipple). Nipples that remain flat or dimple inward during stimulation can make nursing difficult, but exercises or breast shells can help. Ask your caregiver or call La Leche League (see "Resources") or a lactation consultant.

▲ Consider donating your baby's cord blood or banking it for your own family (see page 155).

▲ Know the warning signs of preterm labor (see page 164); premature birth may be preventable if labor is stopped in time.

Third Trimester

MONTH 7

Your baby grows:

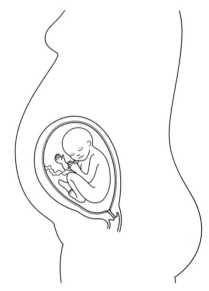

- ▲ The fetus puts on body fat, notices changes in light and dark, and continues to make vigorous movements.
- ▲ Taste buds develop.
- ▲ Chances for surviving a premature birth increase as the fetus grows. Now he is 15 to 17 inches long and weighs between $2\frac{1}{2}$ and 3 pounds.

Month 7

Your body changes:

- ▲ You may experience insomnia, breathlessness, leg cramps, or numb hands or feet, and stretch marks may appear in your skin (see Chapter 5).
- ▲ You may begin to feel Braxton-Hicks contractions (see page 84).

Things to do:

- ▲ Begin taking childbirth classes (see page 123).
- ▲ Investigate child-care possibilities if you plan to go back to work shortly after the birth.

MONTH 8

Your baby grows:

- ▲ As the brain and nerves mature, the fetus responds to sounds and experiences regular periods of sleep and wakefulness.
- ▲ The fetus may assume a head-first position for birth (see page 103).
- ▲ Somersaults decrease after the baby positions herself for birth, but strong kicks continue. You may also feel her hiccups.

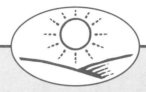

Myths and Facts About Pregnancy and Birth

Trying to figure out whether you're having a boy or girl depending on how you carry can be harmless fun. But believing some common myths about pregnancy and baby care may discourage healthful behaviors or encourage dangerous ones. So discard the myths, and face the facts:

MYTH: The placenta acts as a barrier, protecting your baby against substances that you eat, drink, or inhale.

FACTS: While providing nutrients and water to your baby and transferring your baby's waste products back to you, the placenta actually filters out very little of what you take in.

MYTH: You should toughen up your nipples for breastfeeding by rubbing them with a terry cloth towel.

FACTS: Such preparation does nothing to prevent sore nipples. In fact, harsh rubbing can damage those tender tissues.

MYTH: If you or your partner has twins in the family, you're more likely to see double at your own delivery.

FACTS: The likelihood of having fraternal twins increases only if the mother has twins in her family, is over 35, takes fertility drugs, or has in-vitro fertilization. Twins in your partner's family don't affect your chances. Identical twins are a chance event.

MYTH: An active fetus is more likely to be a boy; a quiet one is more likely to be a girl. You can also tell the baby's sex by the way your fetus lies in the womb or how fast the little heart beats.

FACTS: You have about a fifty-fifty chance of divining the sex by your baby's fetal activity, position, or heart rate in the womb. Since fetal hormones can pass into your blood you might notice sexually determined differences from one pregnancy to the next—*in theory.* In practice, maternal intuition works this way only about 50 percent of the time.

MYTH: Reaching your arms over your head will strangle your baby on her umbilical cord.

FACTS: Well cushioned by amniotic fluid, your baby's cord is unaffected by your arm movements.

MYTH: Eating strawberries or certain other foods during pregnancy can cause birthmarks.

FACTS: Even though some birthmarks look like strawberries, a baby's birthmarks aren't caused by his mother's diet during pregnancy.

MYTH: Your baby will probably stop moving several days before your due date.

FACTS: Healthy babies continue to move until they are born. As you approach your due date, you'll notice fewer somersaults because your baby lacks the room for tumbling. But he should keep right on kicking until birth.

MYTH: If you have a cesarean, your baby will be more likely to have a round head. A vaginal birth will give your baby a long head.

FACTS: At birth, your baby's skull bones will not yet be fused together. To fit through your pelvis, the bones overlap, temporarily elongating your baby's head. This so-called molding depends less on what type of delivery you have than it does on the length of your labor, at what point a cesarean is performed, and your baby's head size compared to your pelvis. Within a few days after birth, the baby's head will assume its normal shape.

MYTH: Fathers rarely experience pregnancy or postpartum symptoms.

FACTS: The century-old term *couvade* refers to symptoms 10 to 35 percent of expectant fathers experience. Fathers' symptoms include indigestion, food cravings, nausea and vomiting, anxiety, insomnia, and weight gain. In addition, some new fathers even suffer postpartum depression.

▲ The fetus is about 16½ to 18 inches long, and weighs between 4 and 5 pounds.

Your body changes:

▲ The top of your uterus reaches your diaphragm, making it easy for you to become short of breath.
▲ You can watch your abdomen move as the fetus shifts in position.
▲ Braxton-Hicks contractions strengthen.

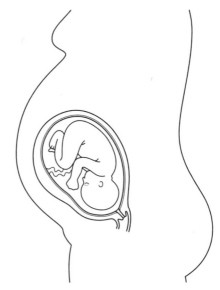

Month 8

Things to do:

▲ Choose a doctor to care for your baby after birth (see page 158).
▲ Begin collecting the clothing and supplies you'll need for your newborn (see page 160); don't forget to buy and install a car seat (see page 160).
▲ Tour the hospital or birthing center where you plan to give birth, and ask about preregistering (see page 130).
▲ Arrange for someone to stay with your older children during the birth.
▲ Make arrangements for postpartum help (see page 159).
▲ Prepare your pet for the new baby (see page 197).

MONTH 9

Your baby grows:

▲ The baby begins gaining your immunities.
▲ The baby's arms and legs are flexed; his head may drop even lower in your pelvis.
▲ The baby's lungs are now mature.
▲ Lanugo (fetal body hair) and cheesy vernix begin to disappear.
▲ The baby assumes his position for birth: more than nine in ten babies are born head down.

▲ The baby gains about a half pound each week. At full term, most babies weigh between 6 and 9 pounds and measure about 20 inches long.

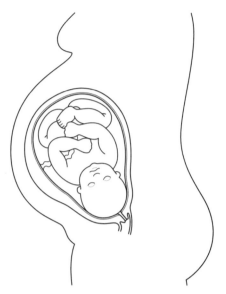

Your body changes:

▲ Shortness of breath will probably disappear once your baby drops lower in the pelvis.
▲ Your navel may stick out as your belly continues to stretch.
▲ Your ankles are probably swollen by the end of the day.

Month 9

▲ Your cervix begins to soften and "ripen." Braxton-Hicks contractions increase.
▲ You can express yellowish colostrum (pre-milk) from your breasts, and a little may leak in your bra (see page 83).

Things to do:

▲ Practice your prepared childbirth techniques.
▲ Buy nursing clothes.
▲ Choose your baby's name (see page 156).
▲ Get instructions from your caregiver about when to call and when to go to the hospital or birth center.
▲ Pack your suitcase for the hospital or birth center (see page 171).
▲ Stockpile frozen dinners for the early postpartum period.

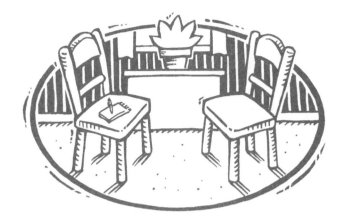

CHAPTER 3

Partners in Prenatal Care

Regular prenatal care, including checkups and tests, offers your baby the best chance to be born healthy. So make an appointment to see the prenatal caregiver you've chosen as soon as you think or know you're pregnant.

During pregnancy you should see your doctor or midwife regularly—probably monthly during your first two trimesters, every two weeks beginning in the seventh or eighth month, then weekly during the ninth month. Women with health problems or high-risk pregnancies usually visit their caregivers more often. Your partner should feel welcome to accompany you to these appointments.

Your First Visit

The first visit, which usually lasts longer than subsequent visits, typically includes a detailed physical examination, a series of tests, a discussion of your medical and family history, and plenty of time for your questions.

Your height, weight, and blood pressure will be measured. In addition to a general physical checkup, your caregiver will perform a thorough pelvic examination. This internal exam includes checking your vagina, rectum, and pelvic organs, and assessing the size and shape of your pelvis. If you like, ask your caregiver to explain each part of the internal exam before performing it. The caregiver will probably use a warmed instrument called a speculum to hold open the vaginal walls, examining the cervix and taking specimens for testing (see below). Wearing a lubricated glove, your caregiver will check your uterus and ovaries by placing two fingers in your vagina while pressing with the other hand on your abdomen. Breathe slowly to stay relaxed. The internal exam should take only a couple of minutes.

Laboratory tests may include—

▲ blood tests to determine your iron or hemoglobin levels, your levels of thyroid-stimulating hormone (TSH), your blood type, and whether you carry the Rh factor (see page 116); whether you have antibodies to rubella (see page 112); if you have syphilis, gonorrhea, or HIV (the virus that causes AIDS); and whether you have been exposed to hepatitis;

▲ a Pap smear, in which cells scraped from your cervix are checked for cervical cancer;

▲ vaginal swab tests for gonorrhea, chlamydia, and bacterial vaginosis; and

▲ a urine sample, to rule out a urinary tract infection and to check for sugar, which may indicate diabetes (see page 104).

Your Due Date

Pregnancy lasts about 38 weeks or 266 days from conception. But your due date gets calculated on the basis of a more easily determined date: the first day of your last menstrual period. This method of figuring a due date gives normal pregnancy a length of 40 weeks, or 280 days from your last period. To figure your due date by this formula, add a year and seven days to the first day of your last menstrual period and then subtract three months.

Before you put a big *X* on your calendar, you should know that your due date is more an educated guess than a firm prediction.

Think instead of your "due month." Though only about 4 percent of babies arrive exactly on their predicted birthdays, about eight out of ten do arrive "at term," or on time: within three weeks before or two weeks after their due dates.

This standard formula to figure the due date assumes a menstrual cycle of 28 days, with ovulation at the midpoint of the cycle. Women with longer or shorter cycles should push their due dates forward or backward by a few days. Consider this, too: Some research suggests that the average length of pregnancy may actually exceed 266 days. One study found that pregnancy lasted an average of 274 days for first-time mothers and 269 days for mothers who had given birth before, 8 days and 3 days longer than suggested by the traditional formula.

Why does your due date matter to your caregiver? About one in ten babies are born preterm (more than three weeks before their due date). A smaller percentage arrive postterm (more than two weeks after their due date). Because babies who are born too early or too late run a higher risk of medical problems, your caregiver may consider intervening if labor begins early or fails to begin by 42 weeks. If you're unsure of the date your last period started you'll probably be encouraged to have an early ultrasound examination (see page 34), which can more closely estimate your due date.

Later Visits

Follow-up visits will usually be shorter than the first visit, but they should always include enough time to discuss your questions and concerns. Think of these appointments as preventive medicine. Most pregnancies progress smoothly. But careful watching may uncover problems that could affect your or your baby's health. Routine follow-up visits typically include—

- ▲ a tummy check to determine the growth of your uterus and the size and position of your baby;
- ▲ measurements of your weight and blood pressure;
- ▲ listening to the fetal heartbeat, either with a special stethoscope called a fetoscope or with an ultrasound device called a Doppler;
- ▲ examination of your urine for sugar, which could indicate diabetes (see page 104), and for protein, which could indicate preeclampsia (see page 115);

▲ a check to see if you are retaining too much fluid, which could also indicate preeclampsia (see page 115);

▲ in the last weeks, internal examinations to check for signs of approaching labor (see page 162).

―――・♥・―――
Building a Working Relationship

You and your caregiver share some common goals: keeping you and your baby healthy and preparing for a good birth. To achieve them, you'll both need to do a lot of talking and listening. These tips should help you do your part:

▲ Keep a running list of questions and bring them with you to your appointments. Encourage your partner to list questions, too, and to accompany you on your prenatal visits.

▲ Whenever your caregiver recommends a procedure, a test, or medication, ask for an explanation of the pros and cons. If you don't understand the explanation, ask for printed information. It may also help to take notes.

▲ Be prepared for a healthy give and take. Clearly communicate your preferences, but remember that you chose your practitioner for her professional experience. Listen to what she has to say.

▲ Talk with your caregiver about what you want to happen at the birth. Birth often presents surprises, so stay flexible. But be sure to discuss beforehand any form of pain relief you think you'd like to use, procedures you'd prefer to avoid, and what should be included in your birth plan (see Chapter 7).

▲ Take good care of yourself, following your caregiver's recommendations on nutrition, supplements, exercise, lifestyle, and medication.

▲ Don't hesitate to call if your questions and concerns can't wait until the next appointment.

―――・♥・―――

Prenatal Tests and Procedures

Your caregiver will probably suggest that you undergo various tests. Some tests are routine; others may be indicated for a particular reason. These tests are described in detail on pages 34 through 42. Don't hesitate to ask why a procedure has been recommended in your case. You may not have many questions about routine procedures such as blood and urine tests. But for screening procedures such as ultrasound and diagnostic tests such as amniocentesis, you'll want to make sure that the test's benefits outweigh any possible risks.

Prenatal Tests You might ask these questions:

Why is this test performed?

How is it done?

What risks, if any, does the test pose to the baby or me?

How experienced are the person doing the test and the laboratory that assesses the result?

How long will it take to get the results?

How dependable are the results?

How might good, bad, or uncertain results change the way we manage my pregnancy?

Could we get the information in another way? How?

How much does the test cost, and will my health plan cover it?

Screening Procedures

The three procedures described here are rarely used by themselves to diagnose pregnancy problems. Instead, the information they provide helps your caregiver decide when further tests are appropriate.

ULTRASOUND   An ultrasound scan uses sound waves to see internal fetal and maternal structures. The ultrasound probe, or transducer, goes on your abdomen, or, very early in pregnancy, inside your vagina. The transducer sends out high-frequency sound waves, whose echoes are changed into a picture on a video screen. The painless procedure usually takes only a few minutes, but it may last up to an hour. Typically, a scan requires a full bladder. Holding your urine may be the most uncomfortable thing about your ultrasound.

Sometimes called sonography, ultrasound is widely considered safe, especially compared to the X-rays it replaced. In fact, no risks of prenatal ultrasound have been found in more than a quarter century of use. But to avoid hazards, experts say that ultrasound should be used in pregnancy only when medically necessary.

Most expectant parents relish the opportunity to see their baby in utero. In fact, a recent study showed that about half of expectant parents would pay for the ultrasound themselves if their health plan didn't cover it. You should know that an ultrasound scan can sometimes spot the baby's genitals. If you prefer to be surprised at the birth by the words "It's a girl" or "It's a boy," be sure to tell your ultrasound technician and caregiver.

Because an early ultrasound can help accurately identify the gestational age of the fetus, most pregnant women now get an ultrasound scan before 20 weeks. After 20 weeks, ultrasound dating is less accurate. Aside from "dating" the pregnancy, other possible medical reasons for prenatal ultrasound include—

- ▲ diagnosing an ectopic pregnancy (see page 21) or miscarriage (see page 21);
- ▲ detecting a multiple pregnancy;
- ▲ checking fetal growth and development;
- ▲ showing the exact position of the fetus and placenta to safeguard them during other prenatal tests, such as chorionic villus sampling (CVS), amniocentesis, or percutaneous umbilical blood sampling (PUBS);
- ▲ diagnosing possible birth defects;
- ▲ assessing fetal well-being in late pregnancy (see page 40);
- ▲ determining the position of the baby;
- ▲ detecting placenta previa, which might necessitate a cesarean delivery (see page 142);
- ▲ identifying a source of bleeding; and
- ▲ measuring the amount of amniotic fluid.

A special type of ultrasound, **Doppler,** has other uses. Prenatal caregivers typically employ a hand-held Doppler device to monitor fetal heart sounds at each prenatal visit after the eleventh week of pregnancy. In late pregnancy, Doppler ultrasound lets a trained technician measure circulation in the placenta and umbilical cord. This technique, called **velocimetry,** can evaluate fetal well-being when the baby seems to be growing slowly or the mother has high blood pressure (see hypertension, page 106).

ALPHA FETOPROTEIN (AFP), TRIPLE SCREEN, OR ULTRA SCREEN TEST

Higher-than-average maternal blood levels of a substance called alpha fetoprotein (AFP), produced in the fetal liver, may indicate the possibility of a neural tube defect, such as spina bifida (open spine) or anencephaly (absence of a brain). Lower than average levels of AFP have been associated with Down syndrome. A simple blood test between about 15 and 18 weeks can help identify whether your baby may have one of these serious birth defects.

By assessing the levels of two other substances in addition to AFP, the so-called **triple screen** is much more accurate in screening for Down syndrome.

The **ultra screen** is a first-trimester screening test for two chromosomal disorders, trisomy 21 (the usual form of Down syndrome) and trisomy 18. This test, which recently completed U.S. clinical trials and is becoming available nationally, involves ultrasound measurement of the fetal neck and a finger-stick test to measure two proteins in the mother's blood. The ultra screen can noninvasively detect 90 percent of fetuses affected with trisomy 18 or 21, but it cannot detect other abnormalities.

Keep in mind that the AFP test, the triple screen, or even the ultra screen, can't diagnose a fetal problem. Abnormal results merely indicate an increased risk of a defect. Further tests are required to confirm the defect or—much more often—to provide reassurance that the fetus is normal.

The most common reason for an abnormal AFP screening result is that the fetus is older or younger than was thought. A multiple pregnancy can also cause a too-high AFP reading. A follow-up ultrasound (see page 34) can accurately estimate fetal age and diagnose twins. It can also detect certain birth defects.

If an ultrasound scan doesn't explain an abnormal test finding, your caregiver may suggest amniocentesis (see page 39), which can accurately diagnose chromosomal problems and neural tube defects. Another option for women who live near major medical centers is a detailed ultrasound by an expert, who can diagnose a neural tube defect through a thorough inspection of the fetal skull and spine.

The AFP screen carries no risk of physical harm, but the extremely high rate of false positives—abnormal results when nothing is wrong—and the tiny percentage of false negatives— normal results when the fetus has a serious problem—may make you opt against it. Women who would never consider amniocentesis or abortion may also decide to skip AFP screening.

But for many pregnant women, AFP or triple screen testing offers these benefits:

▲ For women 35 or older, it may make unnecessary the riskier genetic testing procedure of amniocentesis (see page 39).

▲ For women with no known risk factors for Down syndrome or neural tube defects, the testing can identify affected babies whose conditions would otherwise go unnoticed until birth.

▲ If your baby is found to have spina bifida, early diagnosis will allow your caregiver to arrange the safest possible birth, which might mean an early delivery or a planned cesarean section to minimize trauma to the baby's back and brain. Fetal surgery to reduce paralysis and brain damage may also be possible. Early diagnosis of Down syndrome may help you prepare emotionally for your baby's arrival.

GLUCOSE SCREENING   Between 24 and 30 weeks of pregnancy, most pregnant women are screened for gestational diabetes (see page 104), which could pose risks to you and your baby if it were to remain untreated. To screen for this disease, you'll be asked to give a blood sample an hour after drinking a very sweet drink or eating candy such as jelly beans. If your blood sugar tests high, you will be asked to take a longer and far more accurate test called a glucose tolerance test (GTT). Most women who have high blood sugar levels on the screening turn out to have normal blood sugar levels when they take the more accurate test.

Genetic Tests

Either chorionic villus sampling (CVS) or amniocentesis can take a genetic picture of your fetus, which may reveal genetic defects. You should be counseled before either test about exactly what conditions the laboratory will be testing for. Most women who take these tests receive reassuring results.

CHORIONIC VILLUS SAMPLING (CVS)   Available as an alternative to amniocentesis at some medical centers, CVS allows for the first-trimester diagnosis of genetic disorders. The small number of parents who learn via CVS that their fetus has a severe abnormality therefore have the option of an earlier, safer abortion than would be available after amniocentesis. But, unlike amniocentesis, CVS cannot diagnose neural tube defects. In addition, CVS is slightly more likely than amniocentesis to give uncertain results. So a mother who chooses CVS may still need to follow up with an amniocentesis.

CVS is performed between 10 and 12 weeks of gestation. A sample of the chorionic villi, hairlike extensions from the membrane surrounding the fetus, is removed for analysis. Guided by ultrasound, the doctor passes a needle through the abdomen or inserts a slender catheter through the vagina and cervix to withdraw the chorionic villi from the uterus. Early findings are available within 48 hours, and detailed results after ten days.

Some studies have linked CVS to an increased rate of limb deformities, especially when the test is performed before ten weeks. About one woman in five experiences cramping following the procedure, and about one in three has some bleeding or spotting for a few days. CVS carries approximately a 1.5 percent risk of miscarriage—slightly higher than amniocentesis. The doctor's level of expertise makes a big difference.

Because of the risks of CVS, a woman should consider the test only if her baby faces an increased chance of birth defects—because the mother is older, because a sibling has birth defects, or because either the mother or father has a family history of birth defects. If you have had vaginal bleeding or spotting, if your baby is at high risk for a neural tube defect, or if your doctor lacks experience with the procedure, you might choose a later amniocentesis instead. Genetic counseling can help you make the difficult choice of whether to have CVS or amniocentesis, or whether to forego both tests.

AMNIOCENTESIS   Performed between 14 and 18 weeks by many obstetricians as well as some family practitioners, amniocentesis can be used to diagnose or rule out neural tube defects as well as genetic defects. In the third trimester, amniocentesis can determine if a baby's lungs are mature (see page 165), if a mother has a uterine infection, and if the Rh-positive baby of an Rh-negative mother needs a blood transfusion (see page 116).

Guided by ultrasound, the doctor passes a needle through the abdomen and into the amniotic sac to withdraw a small amount of amniotic fluid. Then the fluid, which contains fetal cells, is cultured and analyzed to detect abnormalities. Genetic results are available in one to three weeks.

Although a local anesthetic numbs the abdomen during the procedure, many women feel cramping or pressure as the amniotic fluid is removed. The risk of miscarriage is about .5 percent, or 1 in 200. As with CVS, the doctor's level of experience makes a big difference. Earlier amniocentesis, performed in the eleventh or twelfth week, can offer earlier results, but also appears to pose a substantially higher risk of miscarriage.

Like CVS, amniocentesis is offered when a mother is older, when she has had a child with birth defects, or when she or the father has a family history of birth defects.

Before planning to have amniocentesis, consider what you will do if your test results bring bad news. Although some women use genetic testing to prepare themselves for the birth of a disabled child, most women who receive bad results with amniocentesis opt to terminate their pregnancies with second-trimester abortions. Genetic counseling can help you with these difficult choices.

PERCUTANEOUS UMBILICAL BLOOD SAMPLING (PUBS)   Also called **cordocentesis,** this new technique allows tests for both infections and genetic diseases to be performed on umbilical cord blood. PUBS is currently available only at large medical centers and can be done only after 16 weeks of pregnancy. The procedure carries a 1 to 2 percent risk of miscarriage. Guided by ultrasound, the doctor inserts a needle through the mother's abdomen and uterus to obtain a sample of blood from the umbilical cord. This takes about ten minutes. Test results are available within two or three days, which allows speedy diagnosis of infections and of conditions such as sickle cell disease and hemophilia. The same technique can be used to give an unborn baby a blood transfusion or to treat an infection.

Optional Diagnostic Procedures

One of two other procedures may be used, in a very rare case, when a caregiver suspects a serious problem with a developing baby. **Embryoscopy** lets a doctor examine an embryo as young as six weeks via a miniature telescope, called an endoscope, inserted through the vagina or via a needle through the abdomen and uterus. To observe a fetus 16 weeks or older, **fetoscopy** employs a tiny telescope typically introduced into the uterus through the abdomen. These procedures should be reserved for situations when their benefits outweigh the added risks of infection and miscarriage.

Late-Pregnancy Tests of Fetal Well-Being

In late pregnancy, you may undergo one or more procedures to determine your baby's condition.

NONSTRESS TEST (NST)   Performed in your caregiver's office or the hospital at the end of pregnancy, this test uses a fetal monitor to measure your baby's heartbeat for a period of 30 to 40 minutes. Just as your heartbeat rises when you exercise, your healthy baby's heart rate should go up with each movement. Occasionally this test is performed with a buzzer, because sound also typically makes a baby's heart beat faster.

Be sure to eat something before you go in for a nonstress test. As you lie on your side, you will be asked to report each movement you feel. In a reactive, or normal, test, the baby's heart rate accelerates about 15 beats per minute for 15 seconds at least twice during a 20-minute period. In a nonreactive test, the baby's heart rate fails to rise, usually because he slept through the test. To encourage movement, you may be asked to drink something sweet or press on your abdomen.

The results of this test help determine if a high-risk pregnancy can continue or if you need other tests, such as a contraction stress test (see below).

CONTRACTION STRESS TEST (CST) OR OXYTOCIN CHALLENGE TEST (OCT)   This late-pregnancy test of fetal well-being assesses how the fetal heart rate responds to uterine contractions. A heartbeat

Danger Signs

These symptoms indicate that you may need immediate medical care. Let your caregiver know right away if you experience any of the following:

Symptom	Possible Problem
Vaginal bleeding	Miscarriage, ruptured tube, preterm labor, or a placental problem, such as placenta previa or placental separation (abruption)
Leaking clear fluid from vagina	Ruptured membranes or preterm labor
Abdominal pain or severe cramping	Ectopic pregnancy, miscarriage, placental separation (abruption), or preterm labor
Frequent vomiting	Dehydration
Sudden puffiness in your face, fingers, or feet	Preeclampsia
Prolonged severe headache	Preeclampsia
Visual disturbances, such as blurred vision, blind spots, or dark spots	Preeclampsia
Pain, burning, or bleeding while urinating	Urinary infection
Painful, hot spot on leg	Blood clot
Vaginal itching or discomfort	Vaginal infection
Fever over 100 degrees Fahrenheit	Infection
Marked change in baby's usual movements	Fetal distress
Severe blow or squeeze to abdomen	Placental separation (abruption)

that stays strong during and after contractions suggests that the baby's placenta is functioning well.

The test is typically performed in the hospital with the mother lying on her side. Because a CST requires a woman to have three 40-second contractions within ten minutes, the test may last for a couple of hours if contractions are infrequent. Contractions are induced by intravenous Pitocin (a synthetic form of oxytocin, the hormone that causes uterine contractions) or by nipple stimulation. Stimulating the nipples causes the release of oxytocin.

A negative CST is good news for you. This means your baby's heart rate remained steady during the contraction. In contrast, a positive CST means the baby's heart rate slowed. A slowed heart rate is a sign that the baby may have trouble coping with labor contractions.

If you are at risk for complications, or if your pregnancy has continued beyond your due date, your caregiver may suggest a CST to determine if your pregnancy can continue, whether your labor should be induced, or whether you need a cesarean.

BIOPHYSICAL PROFILE   This late-pregnancy test of fetal well-being, which can be performed rapidly in your caregiver's office, has two parts and yields five assessments. The profile combines a nonstress test to check the fetal heart rate during movement (see page 40) with an ultrasound scan to show the baby's activity, muscle tone, and breathing movements, and the amniotic fluid volume. A baby in good condition has a reactive nonstress test, moves around, extends and bends its limbs, makes rhythmic breathing movements, and is surrounded by enough amniotic fluid to cushion his umbilical cord. The results of this test can help your caregiver decide whether or not to induce labor if you are at high risk for complications or if your pregnancy has continued beyond your due date. Your caregiver may simplify this test; looking at amniotic fluid volume alone appears to be a good way to diagnose fetal well-being in late pregnancy.

I GET A KICK OUT OF YOU: FETAL MOVEMENT COUNTING   In late pregnancy, most mothers are keenly aware of their babies' typical movement patterns. A healthy baby has several active periods each day. A marked slowdown—or, less frequently, a sudden jump—in your baby's typical activity level may indicate a serious problem and should prompt a call to your caregiver.

To get used to your baby's pattern, pick a time to count your baby's movements every day after your twenty-eighth week. Choose a time when your baby is typically active. When the time arrives, get into a comfortable position. Note how long it takes each day for your baby to make ten separate movements (hiccups don't count). If your baby stays quiet, you may be able to rouse her for the count by poking your abdomen, making a loud noise, or having some juice. Your baby should move at least ten times in two hours. Call your caregiver if your baby is taking longer each day to make ten movements or if she hasn't had an active period within the past several hours.

CHAPTER 4

Healthy Habits

Taking good care of yourself will never win a better payoff than during pregnancy. Not only will you feel better, you'll also be giving your baby every advantage. Now it's more important than ever to pay attention to what you eat, how you move, and the everyday activities you usually take for granted. As you both prepare for parenthood, invite your partner to join you in cultivating healthier habits.

Eating

What you eat during pregnancy provides the building blocks for your baby to grow from a single cell to a cuddly newborn. Your grandmother may have been warned to limit her weight gain to 12 to 20 pounds to avoid a too-large baby and told to restrict her salt intake to prevent preeclampsia (formerly called toxemia). Recent studies indicate that these two pieces of advice caused more problems than they solved.

The Bottom Line: How Much Weight Should You Gain?

It's an important question. Gaining too little weight, especially in the third trimester, puts your baby at risk for being born early.

Gaining too much weight boosts your chance for a cesarean delivery. In 1990, the National Academy of Sciences concluded that babies generally do best when their mothers gain between 25 and 35 pounds. Women who begin pregnancy quite thin should gain more—28 to 40 pounds—while overweight women should gain less—15 to 25 pounds. Expecting twins? Aim to gain between 35 and 45 pounds.

More important than how much you gain is your pattern of gain. In the first trimester, you'll probably gain from two to five pounds. During the last two trimesters, you should gain about a pound a week on average. Tell your caregiver if you experience weight loss or a sudden, dramatic weight gain.

The weight you gain in pregnancy includes four to five pounds of stored fat as well as the baby, uterus, placenta, breasts, and fluids. If you think you can simply bypass those pounds of stored fat, think again. Mother Nature wants you to be able to feed your newborn in case of famine, so your body automatically stores fat in early and mid-pregnancy even if you undereat. During your last trimester, dieting won't work either; the pounds you gain go directly to the baby. So retire any plans to chuck your baby fat until after your baby arrives.

Even then, you'll need to be patient. Although a few lucky women rapidly resume their prepregnancy figures, it's more realistic to anticipate taking several months to lose the weight it will take you nine months to gain.

Where Do All Those Pounds Go?	
baby	7.5 pounds
breasts	1–2 pounds
uterus	2 pounds
placenta	1.5 pounds
amniotic fluid	2 pounds
blood volume	3 pounds
stored fat	4–5 pounds
extra fluid	4–6 pounds
TOTAL	25–29 pounds

A Matter of Quantity

When you're building a baby, you need to eat a bit more—about 300 calories a day—over the 2,000 calories an average-sized non-pregnant woman consumes. This is not the same as eating for two adults. Those 300 extra calories equal a snack: half a sandwich and a glass of low-fat milk, or a glass of orange juice and five or six graham cracker squares.

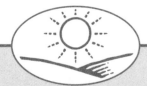

Snack Attack

When you feel hungry between meals, try snacks like these:

▲ dried fruits, such as figs, raisins, and apricots
▲ fresh fruits and vegies, like apples, oranges, and carrot sticks
▲ nuts and seeds, like peanuts, almonds, sunflower seeds, and pumpkin seeds
▲ egg salad, tuna, and peanut butter sandwiches on whole-grain bread or rice cakes
▲ milk shakes or fruit smoothies fortified with dry milk powder for extra calcium
▲ hard-boiled eggs
▲ dry cereal with low-fat milk and raisins or bananas
▲ split pea soup with crackers
▲ custard
▲ plain or fruit-flavored yogurt

No one deserves an occasional treat more than a pregnant mother, but avoid overindulging in cake, candy, cookies, and soda. Instead, get into the habit of spending your extra calories on these all-important nutrients: protein, calcium, and iron (see pages 47 to 53). For nutritious snacks that give you more crackle for the calories, see "Snack Attack."

. . . and Quality

The nutrients you need to build your baby include protein, carbohydrates, fat, vitamins, minerals, and water. Each day of your pregnancy you'll want to take in—

▲ two to three servings of protein
▲ six to eleven servings of carbohydrates
▲ a small amount of fat
▲ four servings of calcium-rich foods
▲ at least four servings of vegetables
▲ at least three servings of fruits

▲ salt to taste
▲ eight cups of liquid

Try to take a broad perspective on eating well. Many women have trouble keeping food down in the first three months, so don't beat on yourself if your diet is less than perfect on any particular day. But if you're not in the habit of keeping a generally balanced diet, do try to change this. Below is more detailed information on the nutrients you and your baby need.

PROTEIN Protein forms the major building blocks for all the baby's tissues as well as your expanding uterus, blood, and placenta. During pregnancy, you'll want to take in at least 60 grams of protein per day (some nutritionists recommend 100 grams a day from the fifth month on). Women expecting twins should aim for at least 100 grams, and women expecting triplets should consume at least 135 grams.

Each of the following foods contains about 15 grams of protein. In addition to a quart of milk, which provides 30 grams of protein, or other foods that contain about the same quantities of both protein and calcium (see "Calcium"), you'll need two or three of these foods each day:

▲ 2 large eggs
▲ 2 to 3 ounces meat, fish, or poultry (a piece the size of a deck of cards)
▲ 2 ounces hard cheese
▲ ½ cup cottage or ricotta cheese
▲ ¼ cup peanut butter, or ½ cup peanuts
▲ ⅔ cup shelled sunflower seeds or almonds
▲ 1 cup cooked beans, split peas, or lentils
▲ ¾ cup cubed tofu (about 6½ ounces)

If you eat little or no meat you can meet your protein needs by eating animal foods such as milk, eggs, and cheese, and by combining such foods, and beans and nuts, with grains. If you are a strict vegetarian—that is, if you get all your protein from plant foods—you should ask your caregiver whether you need supplementary vitamin B_{12}, vitamin D, iron, calcium, and zinc, or consult a nutritional expert or dietitian.

CARBOHYDRATES Starchy foods give you energy for your daily activities and, in combination with other foods, provide some pro-

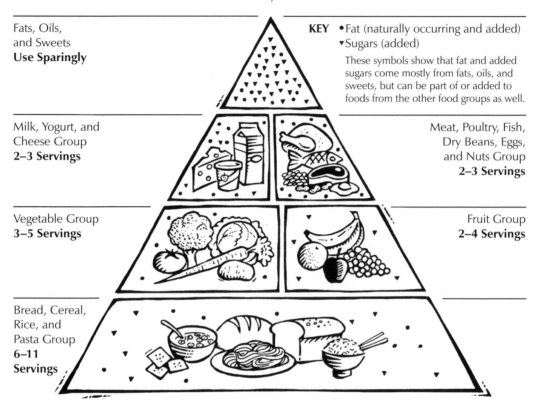

FOOD GUIDE PYRAMID
A Guide to Daily Food Choices

Fats, Oils,
and Sweets
Use Sparingly

KEY • Fat (naturally occurring and added)
▼ Sugars (added)

These symbols show that fat and added sugars come mostly from fats, oils, and sweets, but can be part of or added to foods from the other food groups as well.

Milk, Yogurt, and
Cheese Group
2–3 Servings

Meat, Poultry, Fish,
Dry Beans, Eggs,
and Nuts Group
2–3 Servings

Vegetable Group
3–5 Servings

Fruit Group
2–4 Servings

Bread, Cereal,
Rice, and
Pasta Group
**6–11
Servings**

tein. Whole grains also contain fiber, which can counter constipation. You'll need six to eleven servings a day from these choices:

- ▲ 1 ounce dry cereal
- ▲ ½ cup cooked cereal, such as oatmeal, grits, couscous, or bulgur
- ▲ 1 small waffle or medium pancake
- ▲ ½ cup cooked pasta
- ▲ ½ cup cooked rice
- ▲ 1 slice bread
- ▲ half a bagel, muffin, or roll
- ▲ 1 tortilla or small pita pocket
- ▲ 4 to 6 crackers
- ▲ 2 rice cakes
- ▲ 2 cups cooked popcorn

FATS AND OILS (A LITTLE DAB'LL DO YA)   Fats and oils taste good, satisfy you, and provide the fat-soluble vitamins A, D, E, and K. Your baby also needs essential fatty acids for her growth and development. But ounce for ounce, fats contain more than twice as many calories as proteins and carbohydrates. To avoid gaining too much weight during pregnancy, pay attention to food labels. Try to keep your daily fat intake at or below 30 percent of your daily calories. For the average prenatal diet (2,300 calories), that means a limit of about 70 grams of fat per day. Tasty vegetable sources include olives, avocados, nuts, and seeds.

CALCIUM   The calcium that builds your baby's bones and teeth comes directly from your body's supply. A prenatal diet lacking in calcium may contribute to the later development of a bone-crumbling, crippling condition called osteoporosis. Each day of your pregnancy, you need a bit more calcium than is contained in a quart (4 cups) of milk. Some people can't digest lactose, a sugar found in cow's milk. If milk disagrees with you, drink less at one time, try yogurt or buttermilk, have your milk in cooked foods such as custard or soup, use an over-the-counter product that contains lactase (to predigest the lactose for you), or substitute other high-calcium foods. Caffeine reduces calcium absorption, but you can compensate for this effect by having milk with your coffee. Try to consume four servings daily from these choices:

- 1 cup milk, buttermilk, yogurt, or custard
- $1/3$ cup dry milk powder
- $1\frac{1}{2}$ ounces hard cheese
- $1\frac{1}{2}$ to 2 cups cottage cheese
- $1/2$ cup canned salmon, with bones
- 2 cups cooked soybeans
- 8 ounces tofu
- 1 cup almonds
- $1/4$ cup ground sesame seeds (tahini)
- 2 cups cooked fresh broccoli
- $1\frac{1}{2}$ cups cooked fresh greens, such as kale or collards
- 1 cup soy milk
- 1 cup calcium-enriched orange juice

FRUITS AND VEGETABLES   To get all the vitamins you need, plan to eat at least seven servings of fruits and vegetables each day. One serving equals one-half cup cooked or one cup raw vegetables, a medium piece of fruit, or a 6-ounce glass of juice. Among fruits,

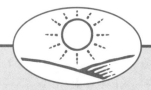

Reading Nutrition Labels

The information provided in Nutrition Facts labels can help you make healthful food choices for yourself and your baby. A label similar to the one shown here for whole wheat bread appears on most packaged food you buy. Government regulations mandate that every label must list—

▲ total calories,
▲ calories from fat,
▲ total fat,
▲ saturated fat,
▲ cholesterol,
▲ sodium,
▲ total carbohydrates (including dietary fiber and sugars),
▲ protein,
▲ vitamin A,
▲ vitamin C,
▲ calcium,
▲ and iron.

This information must be included whether or not the food contains these nutrients. Nutrition Facts labels tell you how much the food contributes to your recommended daily intake of these nutrients ("% daily value"). Labels may include "% daily value" information for other essential vitamins and minerals as well, such as folic acid and vitamin D.

When food shopping, compare products for calorie, fat, sodium, and protein content as well as for vitamins and minerals. Take note of how the standard "serving size" given at the top of the label compares with the amount you usually eat.

The "% daily values" in Nutrition Facts labels are based on a diet of 2,000 calories. During pregnancy, the average woman should consume an additional 300 calories, or about 2,300 total calories per day. Look for foods high in protein, calcium, and iron, but low in fat, to make up the extra calories.

Nutrition Facts

Serving size: 1 slice (36 grams)
Servings per container: 19

Amount per serving

Calories 90
Calories from Fat 10

	% Daily Value*
Total Fat 1.5g	2%
Saturated fat 0g	0%
Cholesterol 0g	0%
Sodium 160mg	7%
Total Carbohydrate 17g	6%
Dietary Fiber 2g	8%
Sugars 3g	
Protein 4g	

Vitamin A	0%	Thiamin	10%
Vitamin C	0%	Riboflavin	4%
Calcium	2%	Niacin	8%
Iron	8%	Folic Acid	6%

* Percent Daily Values are based on a 2,000 calorie diet. Your daily values may be higher or lower depending on your calorie needs:

		Calories	2,000	2,500
Total Fat	Less than		65g	80g
Sat Fat	Less than		20g	25g
Cholesterol	Less than		300mg	300mg
Sodium	Less than		2,400mg	2,400mg
Potassium			3,500mg	3,500mg
Total Carb			300g	375g
Fiber			25	30g

fresh ones are your best choices, followed by those that are frozen, or canned in their own juice. To keep fat intake down and vitamins and minerals up, steam, broil, bake, sauté, or stir-fry your vegetables instead of deep-frying them. Each day, eat:

- ▲ 1 to 2 servings of leafy green vegetables, such as spinach, dark lettuce (not iceberg), Swiss chard, cabbage, broccoli, or collard greens
- ▲ 2 servings of vitamin–C rich foods, such as oranges, grapefruits, cantaloupe, strawberries, peppers, broccoli, cabbage, cauliflower, tomatoes, or potatoes
- ▲ 1 serving of a yellow or orange vegetable or fruit, such as sweet potatoes, winter squash, carrots, pumpkin, cantaloupe, or mango
- ▲ 3 servings of a vegetable or fruit of your choice

SALT Sodium allows your blood volume to expand during pregnancy. So you can salt your food lightly without worry. But a heavy hand with the salt shaker or too many high-sodium packaged foods can contribute to high blood pressure. Beware of heavily salted prepared foods such as luncheon meats, pretzels, chips, pickles, and canned soups.

WATER Drinking liquids helps digestion, gives your baby a soft, fluid cushion, and supports your increased blood volume. Choose plain water, juice diluted with water, milk, soup, and caffeine-free coffee or teas in place of coffee, tea, and soda with caffeine, which drives fluids out of the body. Avoid sugar-sweetened drinks, which are devoid of vitamins and minerals, and artificially sweetened drinks, since the sweeteners may not be good for your baby. For an occasional treat, mix fruit juice with sparkling water. Aim to drink eight cups of liquid each day.

When Cost Is an Issue

If you can't afford to buy the nutritious food you need to eat during pregnancy, you may qualify for several assistance programs sponsored by the federal government. The Supplemental Food Program for Women, Infants, and Children (WIC) provides food vouchers for low-income pregnant and nursing women, and children up to the age of five. In addition, you may qualify for Aid to Families with Dependent Children (AFDC), food stamps, or both. Your caregiver can tell you about these programs or refer you to a social worker.

Other Goodies

VITAMINS   These chemical substances found in foods provide you and your baby the ABCs of good health. Eating a variety of fruits and vegetables will ensure that you have all the letters covered.

Vitamin A   This fat-soluble vitamin helps you resist infection, and possibly cancer, promotes vision, and builds strong tooth enamel. Vitamin A is found in orange and leafy green vegetables (see "Fruits and Vegetables"); liver and other organ meats; butter; and whole and fortified milk. You can't get too much vitamin A in the food you eat, but excessive supplementation can be dangerous for you and your baby.

B vitamins   These water-soluble vitamins help your baby's cells divide and grow. For you they prevent anemia, aid digestion, and promote a sense of well-being. Get your B vitamins from whole grains, organ meats, milk, leafy greens, almonds, and peanuts.

One part of the B vitamin, **folic acid,** or folacin, is particularly important now: Your need for this nutrient doubles during pregnancy. Since a deficiency of folic acid has been linked to serious neural tube defects such as spina bifida, the U.S. government began in January 1998 to require folic-acid enrichment of grain products such as white flour, cornmeal, white rice, and commercial breads and breakfast cereals. For extra protection, most women who are pregnant or trying to become pregnant should also take a vitamin supplement that includes folic acid (see page 5).

Vitamin C   This water-soluble vitamin contributes to sturdy cell walls and a strong placenta, promotes iron absorption, and helps in the formation of a baby's teeth and bones. Vitamin C also aids healing. You should get it daily in fresh fruits and vegetables (see above).

Vitamin D   Your body needs this fat-soluble vitamin in order to use calcium. You can meet your quota each day by spending some time in the sun or by drinking four cups of fortified milk. Other dietary sources include sardines, canned salmon, egg yolks, butter, and liver.

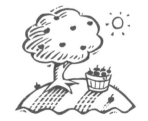

Vitamin E   This fat-soluble vitamin promotes the growth of tissue and the strength of cell walls. Get vitamin E in vegetable oils, whole-grain cereals, meat, eggs, nuts, and seeds.

Vitamin K   Your intestines produce some of this fat-soluble vitamin, which is needed to help blood clot. You can get the rest of the vitamin K you need from green leafy vegetables and vegetable oils.

MINERALS   Pregnancy boosts your needs for two minerals; calcium (see page 49) and iron (below). In addition, you need sufficient sodium (see page 51) and several other important minerals.

Iron   Because your blood volume expands by about 50 percent during pregnancy, you need extra iron to manufacture hemoglobin, the oxygen-carrying protein in blood. Your growing baby also needs to stockpile iron for his first four to six months, the period before he begins to eat regular food.

Because iron is so important in pregnancy, your caregiver may prescribe a supplement. But iron supplements tend to be constipating. To supply iron and prevent constipation, choose foods high in both fiber and iron, such as dried apricots and prunes. Other iron-rich foods include: prune juice, raisins, wheat germ, dried beans, peas, lentils, oysters, almonds, walnuts, tofu, red meats, and organ meats like liver.

Other foods in your diet can affect how well your body absorbs iron. Acidic foods, such as yogurt and citrus fruits, boost iron absorption, but coffee, tea, and antacids all slow the absorption of this mineral. For maximum absorption of iron supplements, take them between meals or at bedtime.

Zinc   This mineral contributes to the development of the fetal nervous system. Because iron supplements can block zinc absorption, try to eat plenty of foods that contain zinc, such as meat, liver, eggs, oysters, beans, nuts, seeds, and whole grains.

Magnesium   Nuts, green vegetables, whole grains, and dried peas and beans are all good sources of this mineral, which helps cell metabolism, activates enzymes, and promotes muscle action.

Phosphorus   This mineral, which helps build strong bones and teeth, can be found in milk, cheese, and meat.

Iodine   Occurring naturally in seafood and seaweed, this mineral is added to most table salt (check for the word "iodized" on the label). Iodine is crucial in producing thyroid hormones; if a mother's diet is deficient in iodine, her baby may be born with a goiter.

Supplements

Healthy eating during pregnancy provides your baby almost everything he needs to thrive. For insurance, many caregivers also prescribe a daily supplement containing iron, folic acid, and several other vitamins and minerals. But remember that no vitamin supplement can make up for a poor diet. And, since excessive supplementation is risky, be sure to ask your caregiver before taking other vitamin supplements in addition to a prenatal multivitamin.

Things You (and Your Baby) Don't Need

When you're pregnant, your baby eats, drinks, and breathes whatever you do. So when you're pregnant, you'll want to be super cautious about what you take in.

ADDITIVES   Eating natural or minimally processed foods lets you avoid the nitrates and nitrites in cured meats, artificial colors, artificial flavors, preservatives such as BHA and BHT, and sodium derivatives like MSG. Although most food additives are safe in small quantities, it can't hurt to be cautious where your baby is concerned.

ALCOHOL   Heavy drinking of beer, wine, or hard liquor is a definite no-no during pregnancy. Alcoholism causes between 2,000 and 12,000 cases of Fetal Alcohol Syndrome (FAS) each year. One of the leading causes of mental retardation, this syndrome also includes heart problems and facial irregularities. Some studies have suggested that even one or two drinks per day during pregnancy can cause later learning and personality problems for a fetus, whose body breaks down alcohol slowly.

Try not to worry about that drink or two you may have had before you realized you were pregnant. Odds are excellent that no harm was done. But because no safe limit for alcohol is known, experts advise women who are trying to get pregnant or who might be pregnant to lay off alcohol completely.

ALFALFA SPROUTS   Hold off on these crunchy salad additions at least until after pregnancy. They can harbor salmonella, a cause of sometimes severe food poisoning.

ARTIFICIAL SWEETENERS   Since experts don't know the effects of these chemicals on the developing fetus, it's probably best to avoid artificial sweeteners such as those found in soft drinks and sugar-free gum. No risks have been attributed to occasional use, though, so don't panic if you discover you ate or drank something sweetened artificially.

CAFFEINE   Caffeine occurs not only in coffee, but also in tea, soft drinks, chocolate, and many over-the-counter medications, such as Excedrin. Some studies have linked heavy caffeine use with miscarriage and low birth weight. In addition, caffeine blocks calcium absorption and acts as a diuretic. Some experts feel pregnant women can safely drink one to two cups of coffee a day. Others advise avoiding caffeine altogether during pregnancy. To avoid headaches from caffeine withdrawal, reduce your intake gradually.

CHEESE AND MILK   Drink and eat only pasteurized milk products, and avoid all soft cheeses such as brie, Camembert, Roquefort, feta, and Mexican varieties. These cheeses, as well as unpasteurized milk and raw foods made from it, can give you a form of food poisoning called listeriosis. Listeriosis can cause miscarriage, premature birth, stillbirth, and meningitis.

DRUGS   Here's a simple rule: take no drugs unless your prenatal caregiver has prescribed or approved them. This includes all over-the-counter drugs as well as prescription medications.

Street drugs such as marijuana, cocaine, heroin, LSD, PCP, speed, and glue can pose a serious threat to your baby, your pregnancy, and your health. Marijuana smoke, for example, is as dangerous to the baby as tobacco smoke (see page 56); in addition, the active component in pot accumulates in the mother's body, increasing the baby's risk. Babies born to mothers who use cocaine are much likelier to be born early and to suffer strokes or brain damage. Cocaine can also cause an expectant mother to hemorrhage. Babies whose mothers use heroin may be born addicted and need to go through withdrawal after birth. Talk to your caregiver—the sooner the better—if you need help getting off any of these drugs during pregnancy. Or contact the chemical dependency unit of a nearby hospital. See "Resources" for toll-free telephone numbers.

FAT SUBSTITUTES   In many people, the new fat substitute Olestra causes cramps, gas, and diarrhea. To make matters worse, Olestra also transports essential fat-soluble vitamins out of your body. Pregnant or not, cut dietary fat some other way.

FISH   Avoid eating swordfish, shark, king mackerel, and tilefish, and limit tuna steaks and canned albacore tuna. Experts are concerned that the mercury content in these fish might cause fetal brain damage. Fish low in mercury include shrimp, canned light tuna, salmon, pollock, and catfish.

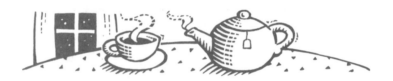

HERBAL TEAS   Most packaged teas are safe, though people allergic to ragweed may prefer to avoid chamomile tea. Herbs that can cause miscarriage include blue and black cohosh, pennyroyal, mugwort, tansy, and slippery elm. Other teas to avoid: goldenseal, sassafras, feverfew, comfrey, yarrow, and kava.

LEAD   Lead pipes or copper pipes soldered with lead can leach the harmful metal into your water, jeopardizing your fetus or young child. To reduce lead in your tap water:

- ▲ If the water hasn't been run for several hours, turn on the tap for five minutes before using the water for drinking or cooking.
- ▲ Use only cold water for drinking and cooking; less lead leaches into it.

Lead can also lurk in some pottery and crystal glassware. Avoid using ceramic or crystal containers to store food and drink unless you know they are lead-free and safe for food.

TOBACCO   The Surgeon General's warning on cigarette packages couldn't be clearer. Smoking by pregnant women raises the risk of fetal injury, premature birth, placental problems, low birth weight and Sudden Infant Death Syndrome. In fact, experts have estimated that smoking during pregnancy is responsible for 10 percent of the infant mortality in the United States. Quitting by the sixteenth week of pregnancy can eliminate the extra risk of having a low-birth-weight baby. Even stopping during your third trimester may improve your baby's growth.

Because the nicotine-delivery systems recommended for other smokers—patches, gum, and nasal sprays—haven't been proven safe for pregnant women, the best approach for quitting is cold turkey. But if you simply can't quit on your own, you may wish to ask your caregiver about nicotine replacement therapy to avoid the other toxic chemicals in smoke and to lower your total nicotine exposure.

If your partner smokes and you don't, your baby still faces a higher risk of being born underweight and of dying of Sudden Infant Death Syndrome (SIDS). Encourage your partner to quit smoking or to smoke outside. The bottom line: If you're pregnant or have a new baby, avoid smoking and breathing smoky air.

RAW OR UNDERCOOKED MEAT, FISH, AND EGGS   Raw or undercooked meat, poultry, and fish can harbor salmonella, listeria, and toxoplasma, microorganisms that can make you very sick and threaten your baby. So walk past the oyster bar and skip the fish sushi, sashimi, rare hamburgers, and steak tartare. Use separate cutting boards for meat and vegetables, and wash your hands and kitchen surfaces thoroughly after handling raw meat. Even raw or lightly cooked eggs in eggnogs, soft-boiled or runny scrambled eggs, cookie dough, Caesar salads, or homemade mayonnaise sometimes contain salmonella—so, to be safe, eat only well-cooked eggs.

Exercising

Exercising for just half an hour most days of the week can give a person a longer life, a healthier heart, improved overall fitness, better sleep, a perkier mood, and an energy boost. During pregnancy, regular exercise offers all these benefits and then some. For one thing, exercise can ease some of pregnancy's common discomforts, such as backache, fatigue, constipation, swelling, leg cramps, and varicose veins. For another thing, exercise will help you build stamina for coping with labor, birth, and the demands of a new baby.

Some research has suggested that exercise may even shorten labor or make premature delivery less likely. And a recent study found that newborns whose mothers swam, ran, or took aerobics classes during pregnancy were less fussy and more alert than other infants. The bottom line is clear: Regular exercise benefits most mothers and babies. It's safe, too, with only a few simple precautions.

Exercising Safely for Two

In several key ways, pregnancy changes your response to exercise. If you had a regular exercise routine before getting pregnant, you may need to alter it to accommodate these changes.

Pregnant women need more oxygen, for example, so you may become breathless when you move too fast. Though pregnancy boosts your body's self-cooling ability, getting overheated—especially during the first trimester—can raise the risk of birth defects. After the fourth month of pregnancy, exercising while lying flat on your back cuts off your circulation and slows your heartbeat, depriving your baby of oxygen. Standing still for long periods can have the same bad effects. As your belly grows, your center of gravity shifts, threatening your balance. Finally, the pregnancy hormones that relax your connective tissues can make injury more likely.

To exercise safely for two, the American College of Obstetricians and Gynecologists offers these tips:

▲ If you're being treated for a medical condition that can make exercise risky (see page 59), check with your caregiver before beginning or continuing any exercise program.

▲ Stop exercising when you get tired.

▲ Avoid becoming overheated. Drink plenty of water before and during exercise; dress in layers; and stay inside on hot, humid days.

▲ To promote blood flow and oxygen delivery to your baby, avoid prolonged periods of standing still throughout pregnancy, and avoid lying on your back after your fourth month.

▲ Choose activities that don't challenge your balancing skill or risk injury to your abdomen.

▲ If you exercise regularly, you may need to exceed the 300 calories that the average pregnant woman adds to her diet.

Be sure to ask your doctor for specific exercise instructions if you're being treated for a medical condition, such as high blood pressure, diabetes, heart disease, or a thyroid condition. And don't force yourself to exercise if you feel too sick to do so during the first few months.

Your caregiver may tell you to avoid exercise if—

▲ you experienced preterm labor contractions during this or a previous pregnancy,

▲ you've had persistent vaginal bleeding,

▲ you have a cerclage (a stitch to keep your cervix closed during pregnancy), or

▲ your fetus isn't growing properly.

If your caregiver advises you not to exercise, ask exactly what you can and can't do. Exercise prohibitions usually refer to aerobic activities such as walking, jogging, and sports. But, with the exception of squatting, you should be able to practice the simple techniques for moving comfortably and relaxing described later in this section (pages 60 to 71). Ask, too, whether it's safe for you to practice Kegels, gentle toning exercises to strengthen the pelvic floor and abdominal muscles (see page 63).

Aerobic Exercise

With your caregiver's okay, you can do aerobic exercise—activities that raise your heart rate and condition your lungs—throughout pregnancy. Brisk walking provides these benefits with no risk.

Do you prefer high-intensity exercise? Jogging and aerobic dancing will probably get harder to do as your pregnancy progresses. If you normally engage in these challenging activities, don't be surprised to find yourself decreasing your workout intensity as your pregnancy advances. Pregnant joggers, for example, sometimes find themselves slowing to a walk to combat fatigue. If you can't carry on a conversation while you exercise, you need to slow down or substitute a different activity. Swimming may be ideal. Not only does your weight gain increase your buoyancy, but the water pressure in the pool also reduces swelling. Another good choice is a stationary bike, which supports you and reduces pressure on your joints.

Because of looser ligaments, changes in balance, and extra weight, pregnant women are more prone to knee and ankle injuries and falls. Treating a fracture is complicated during pregnancy, so postpone hazardous activities such as waterskiing, diving, snowmobiling, horseback riding, and contact sports like basketball and football until after the baby comes. Because skiers risk dangerous falls, especially in the last trimester, stay on easy slopes if you ski. And be sure to wear a helmet if you bike.

For land exercise, wear a supportive bra and well-padded shoes. If you haven't exercised regularly before pregnancy, start with 10- to 15-minute sessions and add a few minutes each week. To avoid injury, warm up for five minutes before exercising and cool down by slowing your pace for five minutes afterward. Slow down or switch activities as soon as you begin to feel tired. Drink plenty of water before and after exercising. And stop exercising immediately if you experience any of these symptoms:

- ▲ breathlessness
- ▲ dizziness
- ▲ headaches
- ▲ muscle weakness
- ▲ nausea
- ▲ chest pain or tightness
- ▲ more than four uterine contractions in an hour, or contractions that persist beyond one hour
- ▲ vaginal bleeding or leaking fluid

Moving Comfortably

The shifting center of gravity and relaxed joints of pregnancy can make it hard to stand, sit, and lift comfortably. Paying more attention to your posture and movements should help reduce backaches and other common pregnancy aches and pains (see Chapter 5).

STANDING TALL   As your abdomen grows, the curve of your back naturally increases. The extra weight you carry in front may make you want to let it all hang out. Unfortunately, doing so can give you a backache as your back muscles strain to keep your body balanced. Instead, use your abdominal muscles to keep your lower back as straight as possible.

Follow these steps to good posture:

▲ Hold your head high.

▲ Draw your shoulders down and back.

▲ Pull in with your tummy muscles.

▲ Tuck in your buttocks.

▲ Relax your knees a little.

▲ Support your body weight evenly on both feet, preferably in flat or low-heeled shoes.

▲ Check yourself in a mirror until good posture becomes second nature.

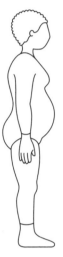 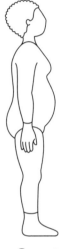

Incorrect   Correct

DON'T JUST STAND THERE, DO SOMETHING   Standing can give you a backache if the extra weight in front pulls you into poor posture. If your back hurts when you stand, straighten it by correcting your posture or by lifting one foot onto a footrest.

Standing still also slows the return of blood from your legs to your heart and head. This isn't good for your baby, and it can make you feel dizzy. Moving around a bit stimulates the upward blood flow.

SITTING PRETTY   Sitting still for a long time can also cause blood to pool in your lower body. To prevent this, avoid crossing your legs at the knees for long periods and do ankle circles to boost your circulation. Putting a pillow behind your back and resting your feet on a footrest will probably make you feel more comfortable in a chair. Or try sitting on the floor, tailor style, with your legs crossed at the ankles. On a long drive, stop every hour to stretch your legs and walk around.

UPLIFTING EXPERIENCES   To avoid injuring your back, let someone else do the heavy lifting while you're pregnant and for at least six

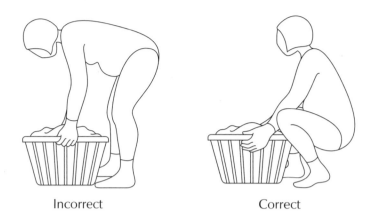

Incorrect   Correct

weeks afterward. If you need to lift something, use your upper arm and thigh muscles instead of your low back muscles to do the work. Stand close to the object, squat to pick it up, and avoid twisting your body as you lift. If you can't do a full squat (see below), bending your knees even a little will help your back.

SQUATTING Besides preventing backaches, squatting offers another major benefit. This position also opens your pelvic bones to the widest diameter, making it an ideal position for the pushing stage of labor. The birthing beds in many hospitals have squatting bars that offer support for women who want to squat while they push. Squatting may be difficult and tiring at first, but daily practice should make it easier.

Some women should skip this exercise. Don't squat if the position hurts your hips, pubic joint, knees, or ankles. If you have risk factors for preterm labor (for example, if you have given birth prematurely; if you are pregnant with multiples; or if you have a cerclage, or stitch to keep your cervix closed), the bearing-down involved in squatting may not be a good idea. Check with your caregiver first.

To practice squatting—

▲ Begin with your feet shoulder-width apart and pointed out at a slight angle; you may need to move your feet a little farther apart to get down.

▲ Bend your knees and squat, resting your weight on your heels as well as your toes.

▲ It may help you to hold on to a chair, to lean back against a wall, or to wear shoes with slight heels.

▲ Hold the position for 15 seconds at first; gradually work up to squatting for 60 to 90 seconds at a time.

▲ Rise slowly, without bouncing.

▲ Repeat five times each day.

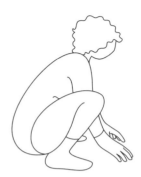

RISE AND SHINE   Simply getting out of bed in the morning may be a challenge as your pregnancy advances. What may come naturally when you aren't pregnant—a sit-up with straight legs—now strains your overworked abdominal and back muscles. Instead, roll over onto your side, bending your hips and knees. Then use your arms, not your abdominal muscles, to lift yourself into an upright position. If you're close to the edge of the bed, drop your legs over the edge to help lift the upper half of your body.

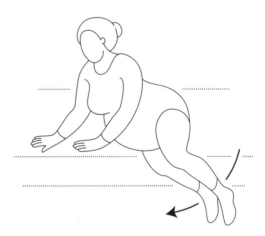

Toning the Muscles That Count Most

Two sets of muscles—the pelvic floor muscles and the abdominal muscles—come under extra stress during pregnancy and birth. Giving these muscle groups special attention every day will pay off during pregnancy, birth, and afterwards.

KEGEL EXERCISES   The pelvic floor muscles, which support your pelvic organs like a sling, extend from your pubic bone in front to your tail bone behind. These muscles, which stretch to allow birth, can sag during pregnancy thanks to the increasing weight of the uterus and the relaxing hormones of pregnancy.

Kegel exercises, named for the doctor who developed them in the 1940s, allow the pelvic floor muscles to stretch more easily during birth and to recover faster afterward. Kegel exercises may also be helpful in preventing future prolapse, or dropping, of the uterus. The regular practice of Kegels can also prevent or reverse mild urinary incontinence (see page 90). Best of all, Kegels enhance your sexual enjoyment because they strengthen the muscles you use in intercourse and orgasm. Once you learn to do Kegels, you can practice anywhere and in any position—in the shower, behind the wheel of your car, in line at the grocery store, at your desk, and in bed with your partner.

Here's how to Kegel:

▲ Begin in a comfortable position, with your legs uncrossed.

▲ Breathing in a relaxed way, place your hands on your abdomen to remind you to keep your abdominal muscles loose.

▲ Draw your pelvic floor muscles inward and upward as if you were squeezing a tampon. Avoid contracting your buttocks, thighs, or stomach muscles. To be sure you're isolating the pelvic floor muscles, put a finger or two in your vagina, then squeeze as if you're trying to stop the flow of urine. Your fingers should feel pressure from the side walls of your vagina.

▲ Hold for a slow count of three; eventually build up until you can hold each squeeze for 10 to 20 seconds.

▲ Release slowly and relax for several seconds, then repeat.

▲ Aim to do 60 to 80 Kegels each day, 10 at a time.

▲ When you urinate, notice how you reverse the Kegel exercise by releasing the pelvic floor muscles and bearing down. You'll do that same reverse Kegel, releasing and bearing down, when you push out your baby.

Kegel exercises can help you learn to relax as well as strengthen your pelvic floor muscles. In late pregnancy, you may wish to add perineal massage (see page 141) to your pelvic floor muscle exercise routine.

ABDOMINAL EXERCISES Your abdominal muscles must expand enormously to make room for your growing uterus, then contract during delivery to push out your baby. Though these muscles feel tight as pregnancy progresses, they're really stretched. In fact, the lengthwise bands of muscle that run down the front of the abdomen actually separate in as many as two out of three pregnant women. You might notice a muscle separation in late pregnancy if your tummy bulges like the roof of a house when you have a bowel movement or climb out of the bathtub. This painless separation can strain your lower back by failing to maintain your good posture.

During pregnancy, you can prevent or minimize muscle separation by breathing out whenever you exert yourself; this decreases intra-abdominal pressure. Also, avoid exercises and actions that strain your back and abdominal muscles. No-nos include double-leg lifts, straight-leg sit-ups, and straight-leg sit-backs.

In contrast, the pelvic tilt does your back good. This gentle exercise strengthens your abdominal muscles, encouraging good posture. Try the pelvic tilt in several positions, including on your back if you are less than four months pregnant. After your fourth month, perform the pelvic tilt in the other positions only. Do five to ten pelvic tilts a day.

You can correct an abdominal separation after the birth by doing another simple exercise; see page 189.

Back-lying pelvic tilt

▲ Lie on your back with your knees bent and your feet flat on the floor.

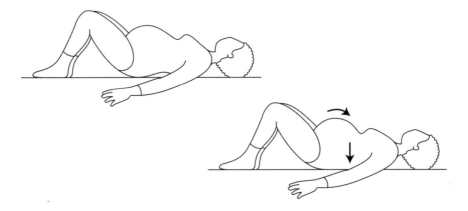

▲ Flatten your waist against the floor by contracting your abdominal muscles.

▲ Hold for a count of five as you breathe out.

▲ Inhale as you relax.

Hands-and-knees pelvic tilt

▲ Get on your hands and knees on the floor, your knees shoulder-width apart.

▲ Begin with your back flat, not curved toward the floor.

▲ Tighten your abdominal muscles to arch your lower back like an angry cat.

▲ Hold for a count of five, while breathing out.

▲ Inhale as you relax to the straight-back position.

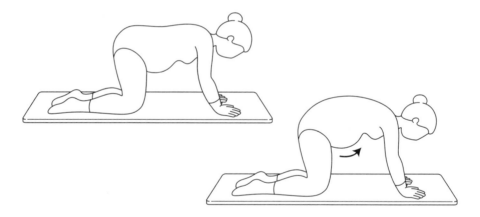

Leaning pelvic tilt

▲ Stand about one foot away from your kitchen counter or a chair that won't slide. The top of the chair or counter should fall between your navel and your pubic bone.

▲ Put your hands on the counter or chair.

▲ With your knees slightly bent, tighten or pull in your abdominal muscles and draw your buttocks forward as if you were pulling a tail between your legs.

▲ Hold for a count of five, while breathing out.

▲ Inhale as you relax back to your original position.

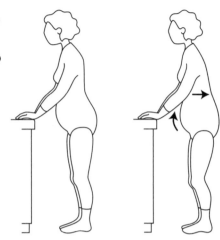

Standing pelvic tilt

▲ Stand with your shoulders and buttocks against a wall, your feet a couple of inches from the wall, and your knees slightly bent.

▲ Pull in your abdominal muscles until your waist touches or nearly touches the wall.

▲ Hold for a count of five, while breathing out.

▲ Inhale as you relax back to your original position.

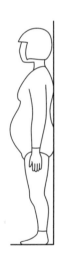
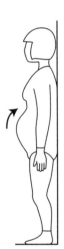

Relaxing

Releasing unnecessary muscle tension can ease some of pregnancy's discomforts, reduce labor pain, and provide energy for taking care of your baby. If you're worried about birth or becoming a parent, relaxation may also calm you. Even if you have no worries, relaxation is good practice for quieting yourself before trying to cope with a squalling newborn.

GETTING STARTED   Many people raise their shoulders when they get tense; others grit their teeth, clench their fists, or get head-aches. As you learn to relax, try to let go of tension in your typical trouble spots.

Most people find that they begin to relax as soon as they slow down their breathing. Simply sighing or yawning a few times can bring on a feeling of peace and restfulness. Try it.

Begin your relaxation practice in a quiet room or while listening to some peaceful music. As you improve at relaxing, you should be able to relax even under noisier conditions.

Start your relaxation practice in the position most comfortable for you. You may prefer lying on your side, with your limbs slightly bent and supported by pillows. Or try reclining in a comfortable chair, with your feet supported on a hassock and your back, arms, and head resting on pillows. Once you can relax in one of these positions, try practicing in a regular chair, letting your head and arms rest on a pillow placed on a table in front of you. As you get even more skilled, try relaxing unnecessary muscle tension in the shower or tub, while standing and leaning, while walking, and even while driving.

WHATEVER CALMS YOU DOWN   A childbirth class should include guided instruction on several types of relaxation, but you can enjoy the benefits of relaxation even before you begin classes. Since each person likes to relax in a different way, experiment with several different methods. Then choose your favorites, and practice daily.

Record the instructions below on an audio tape, or have your partner read them very slowly, giving you plenty of time to respond. After you've heard the instructions, your partner can check to see if your muscles are soft and relaxed or hard and tense. When gently lifting your limbs to check for relaxation, your partner should support you completely and use words or phrases that encourage you to relax, such as *soft, warm, loose, limp noodle, rag doll, let go,* or *release.* To avoid dizziness, always rise slowly after a relaxation session.

General relaxation

▲ Stretch your legs, pointing your toes up toward your face and your heels down. As you breathe out, relax your legs.

▲ Contract your buttocks muscles. As you breathe out, relax them.

▲ Stretch your entire spine. As you breathe out, relax.

▲ Stretch your hands towards your feet. As you breathe out, relax your arms.

▲ Shrug your shoulders toward your ears. As you breathe out, relax, dropping your shoulders.

▲ Make a frown. As you breathe out, relax your facial muscles.

Passive relaxation

▲ As you breathe slowly, let your eyes close. Feel relaxation around your eyes.

▲ Allow the feeling of relaxation to spread from your eyes to your forehead . . . to your scalp . . . all around the back of your head . . . to your ears and temples . . . to your cheeks and nose . . . to your mouth.

▲ Relax your jaw muscles, letting your mouth open slightly.

▲ Relax the muscles in your neck and let the feeling of relaxation spread down into your shoulders.

▲ Now let the relaxation radiate down your arms . . . to your elbows . . . your forearms . . . your wrists . . . your hands. Relax each of your fingers.

▲ Send relaxation down into your pelvis, and allow your buttocks to let go.

▲ Feel the sensation of release move down your thighs, to your calves . . . your ankles . . . your feet . . . and your toes.

▲ Keep breathing slowly. Enjoy the feeling of release, letting go a little more with each exhaled breath.

Relaxation through self-suggestion

▲ In a comfortable position, repeat the following phrases to yourself as you let each part of your body become more relaxed:

▲ My right arm is warm and heavy.

▲ My left arm is warm and heavy.

▲ My right leg is warm and heavy.

▲ My left leg is warm and heavy.

▲ My trunk is warm and heavy.

▲ My heartbeat is slow and regular.

▲ My breathing is slow and regular.

▲ My forehead is cool.

▲ I am relaxed and at peace.

Countdown to relaxation

▲ Imagine yourself on an escalator, beginning on the fifth floor, being carried down to a state of deeper and deeper relaxation.

▲ Breathe out slowly as you release tension in your head, face, and neck. Feel yourself being carried down to the fourth floor.

▲ As you descend to the third floor, breathe out as you relax your shoulders, back, arms, and hands.

▲ Keep breathing, relaxing more with each exhaled breath. Relax your pelvis and buttocks as you descend to the second floor.

▲ Breathe out as you relax your hips, knees, thighs, ankles, and feet. You have now reached the ground floor, a state of deep relaxation.

Relaxation through meditation

▲ Deeply relax all your muscles from your feet up to your face.

▲ Become aware of your breathing, concentrating on a single word or phrase of your choice each time you exhale.

▲ Let yourself relax. If your mind wanders, gently bring your concentration back to your focal word or phrase as you breathe out.

▲ After 15 minutes or so of concentration, sit quietly for several minutes with your eyes closed. Then slowly open them.

Special-place relaxation

▲ After becoming relaxed with one of the methods above, continue resting with your eyes closed.

▲ Think of a beautiful, safe place where you feel calm and peaceful.

▲ First, imagine everything you can see as you turn slowly in a circle. What shapes, colors, and patterns appear to you?

▲ Now listen to all the sounds you can hear, including the sound of your own relaxed breathing.

▲ Allow yourself to feel the pleasant temperature and the surface under your feet. What else do you feel?

▲ Smell any fragrances and recall any tastes associated with your special place.

▲ Allow yourself enough time to enjoy all the good feelings of being in your special place.

Relaxation through breathing

▲ Sit comfortably. As you inhale, think "I am . . . ," and, as you exhale, think "relaxed." Repeat several times, relaxing more with each breath.

▲ With each inhaled breath, try to locate tension somewhere in your body. As you exhale, release the tension. Repeat several times.

▲ As you breathe in, think of taking in oxygen and energy. As you breathe out, focus on releasing tension or pain. Repeat several times.

Adapting Your Lifestyle

Having a baby changes your life in ways you can hardly imagine beforehand. But even before your baby arrives, you'll probably need to make at least a few lifestyle adjustments. For many women, these changes are minor: putting your feet up most evenings instead of going out, for example. Other women find pregnancy trying because medical restrictions severely limit their work or play routines. The following sections cover lifestyle changes that most pregnant women must make. Be sure to ask your own caregiver for individual advice.

Keeping Cool

A prolonged fever that raises your body temperature over 102 degrees Fahrenheit can pose a serious threat to your fetus, especially during the first trimester. Maternal overheating during early pregnancy has been linked to spinal abnormalities and other serious birth defects. So caregivers warn pregnant women to avoid hot tubs, steam rooms, saunas, very hot baths and showers, tanning salons, and workouts in very hot weather.

But it takes time for your temperature to rise to 102 degrees. If you're a determined sauna or hot tub fan, ask your caregiver whether it's safe to limit your exposure to ten minutes, or to take your temperature before exposure and get out when your body temperature has risen one degree. In a hot tub you can keep your body temperature from rising too high too fast by keeping your arms and shoulders out of the water.

You needn't worry about using your electric blanket or about the fever of a minor illness, though you should call your caregiver if you run a fever of 100 degrees or higher. Nor must you shiver in your shower or bath. Water as warm as 100 degrees won't raise your body temperature for the prolonged periods that cause fetal problems.

Resting

When you're pregnant, you need more rest than usual. Unfortunately, as pregnancy progresses, you may have trouble sleeping through the night. Most women find themselves waking repeatedly to find a comfortable position, to adjust the pillows, or to urinate.

To minimize wakings, avoid coffee, tea, and cola late in the day. In addition to keeping you awake, the caffeine in these drinks acts as a diuretic, increasing urination.

Exercising for 30 minutes a few days a week can also promote better sleep. So can extra pillows, including special pregnancy pillows.

If a decent night's sleep continues to elude you, try to make up some of the lost sleep with a daily catnap. Even if you can't nap, merely putting up your feet at lunchtime or during an afternoon break should help you feel a bit more rested. Try also the suggestions for relaxation on pages 67 to 71.

Sex

Your desire for sex may rise or fall during pregnancy. In the early months, for example, your interest may drop because of fatigue, nausea, or breast tenderness. Or you may find yourself more interested in sex because you no longer have to worry about trying to get pregnant. Likewise, as pregnancy advances, you may continue to enjoy sex, or you may find trying to get close more comically awkward than passionate.

Your partner, too, may have changing or conflicting feelings about sex during pregnancy. Excitement about your enlarged breasts and belly may stimulate his sexual desire, for example, but an unrealistic fear of hurting the fetus could stifle it. Some men—some women, too—initially find it difficult to reconcile their sexual ideal of a slender, adolescent female figure with a more mature, maternal sexual image. This problem may resolve itself with time and discussion or may require professional counseling.

If your pregnancy proceeds normally, you and your partner can probably have sex in any way you both find fun, as long as your bag of waters (which protects you and the baby from infection) remains intact. Intercourse doesn't hurt the fetus; cushioned by amniotic fluid, your baby is also protected by the mucus plug that lines the cervix and by the amniotic membranes. In late pregnancy, you may need to experiment to find comfortable positions for intercourse. And you'll definitely need to communicate about what you each need, enjoy, and desire.

There are four important exceptions to the "anything goes" rule:

▲ Because new partners introduce you to increased risks of sexually transmitted diseases (see page 112), monogamy is critical for your health as well as your baby's.

▲ Your sexual partner should not blow into your vagina. This could cause a life-threatening air bubble to enter your bloodstream through your dilated veins.

▲ Anal intercourse followed by vaginal sex could introduce infection into your bloodstream, threatening you and your baby.

▲ Stop having sex and consult your caregiver if you notice signs of preterm labor (see page 164).

If your pregnancy is considered high-risk—perhaps because you had previous miscarriages or a premature delivery, or you are currently expecting more than one baby—ask your caregiver for individual guidelines on exactly what you can and cannot do. For example, should you avoid all sexual contact or just vaginal intercourse? Throughout pregnancy or just for the first three or last three months? Couples who should not have vaginal sex can stimulate each other with their hands and mouths, enhancing their sexual repertoires in the process.

Aside from the obvious changes, pregnancy brings some others that may affect your sexual comfort and pleasure. You should know that—

▲ During pregnancy and for six weeks afterward, douching may cause vaginal infection (see page 97) and more serious problems.

▲ Colorless vaginal discharge normally increases during pregnancy.

▲ Vaginal yeast infections, which cause discomfort and itching, are common during pregnancy (see page 97).

▲ Uterine contractions following orgasm are common and don't endanger a healthy fetus. But call your caregiver if contractions persist for more than an hour.

▲ Urine leakage during sex is common during pregnancy; if it happens to you, do more Kegels (see page 63).

▲ Swollen tissues can cause spotting after sex. You may want to experiment with positions. For example, when you're on top, you can avoid deep penetration. Report persistent spotting to your caregiver, especially if it is accompanied by cramping, and call your caregiver immediately if you experience any significant bleeding or fluid leakage.

Staying Safe at Home, Inside and Out

During pregnancy, home safety means paying more careful attention to the air you breathe and the cleaning supplies you use, as well as paints, pesticides, hair-care products, and even the family pet.

 CLEAN AIR   The air you breathe shouldn't make you and your baby sick. Avoid inhaling secondhand tobacco smoke, as well as the fumes from kerosene space heaters, paints, paint removers, insecticides, weed killers, automobiles and trucks, power lawn mowers and leaf blowers, and chemical cleaning supplies. Pitch aerosol containers, and check the labels on all your cleaning agents. If the instructions caution against skin contact or recommend using only in a well-ventilated area, find a safer product to use instead.

You needn't panic about an occasional whiff of something toxic. But let your nose be your safety guide. Ventilate any room where you smell fumes, or remove yourself from the affected area.

SKIN AND HAIR CARE   Read the labels on your hair-care products, too, or ask your beautician which hair coloring products are safest to use during pregnancy. Many hair dyes contain coal tar, which may cause cancer or chromosomal damage. The less contact between these substances and your scalp, the better. It's probably a good idea to avoid hair dyes altogether during the first trimester. And check any home hair-bleaching or waxing products for warnings.

MICROWAVE OVEN   Don't stand in front of it while it's on, and repair or replace the oven if the door seal is loose.

PETS   To stay on the safe side, avoid taking in a stray animal during pregnancy.

If you have a **cat,** you should know about toxoplasmosis. This infection, caused by protozoa that lurk in cat feces as well as undercooked meat (see page 57), affects most adults mildly but can cause serious damage to a developing fetus. You needn't give away a beloved animal; just observe these simple safety precautions during pregnancy:

- ▲ Let someone else clean the cat litter box.

- ▲ Keep your cats indoors if possible.

- ▲ Avoid feeding your cats raw meat.

- ▲ Wear gloves when gardening to avoid contamination with cat feces.

- ▲ Wash garden vegetables very carefully to remove all soil.

- ▲ Keep sandboxes covered, and wash your toddler after he plays in the dirt or sand.

Mid-pregnancy is a good time to attend obedience training with your **dog,** if you haven't already done so. When you take her out, notice how she reacts to babies. Most dogs adapt quickly to having a new baby around the house and act loving and protective. But an animal that responds aggressively when approached, while eating, or when startled will need extra supervision around a baby. If necessary, get your dog used to a muzzle or leash well before the birth. Shortly before the baby arrives, have your dog sit while you practice such baby-care tasks as diapering, using a doll; give your dog a treat afterward. You should also let your dog sniff the baby's new clothes and furniture.

After the birth, have your partner present for the dog's inspection a blanket or piece of clothing used by your newborn. And, just before you and your newborn arrive home from the hospital or birth center, have someone feed the dog so she will be calm.

Turtles and lizards can carry salmonella, which can seriously threaten you and your developing baby. So wear gloves when you clean the tank, handle your reptile, or change his water.

Traveling Safely

With a few adaptations, such as avoiding high altitudes in late pregnancy, you can travel safely. But be sure to keep eating well and drinking enough water. Choose bottled water or boil tap water for 15 minutes, if you're in a country where the drinking water may be contaminated. When you travel avoid standing or sitting still for too long. Check with your caregiver about the best forms of travel and time windows for traveling in your specific situation.

BY CAR You can drive throughout your pregnancy until labor begins, as long as you can still fit behind the wheel. To avoid sitting still too long, though, schedule hourly stops to get out and stretch your legs. Occasionally, a pregnant woman may have to curtail driving due to dizzy or fainting spells or severe nausea.

Always fasten your seat belt. Contrary to popular belief, seat belts won't harm your fetus or breasts. Unbuckled, you and your fetus face a much greater risk of dying in an accident. Here's the best way to wear your seat belt:

▲ Sit up straight so the belt stays below your belly.

▲ Adjust the lap belt snugly below your belly and across your upper thighs.

▲ Position the shoulder strap tight across your shoulder and between your breasts; place it above your belly in late pregnancy.

▲ Seek medical attention quickly if you are in a motor vehicle accident, no matter how minor. Though your baby is well protected, even a mild collision could separate the placenta from the uterus and threaten the baby.

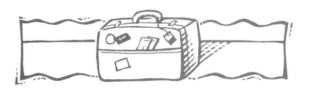

BY PLANE Unless your pregnancy is complicated by heart disease, respiratory problems, or a blood disorder such as sickle cell disease, you'll probably get the green light to fly until your last month of pregnancy. Some caregivers discourage flying in the last trimester for women with hypertension, preeclampsia, or diabetes; women who have previously given birth prematurely; and women who are expecting more than one baby. If you have a condition requiring medication and your caregiver okays a lengthy plane trip, ask about adjusting your medication schedule to accommodate the time change.

Because some airlines restrict travel by obviously pregnant women without written medical approval, ask your caregiver for a medical certificate if you plan a plane trip during your last trimester. To avoid unnecessary radiation, bypass the electronic security scan in favor of a personal check by a female security guard.

Reserve an aisle seat so you'll feel free to get up to walk for about ten minutes every hour. If possible, elevate your feet by stretching them out on an empty seat next to you, or setting them down on a makeshift footrest. This will be easier if you sit in the bulkhead section, where there is extra leg room. Wear comfortable clothes, and be sure to pack some loose-fitting shoes, because your feet may swell. The air on an airplane is very dry, so you may want to tote a thermos of cold water or iced herbal tea. You can minimize the gas that plagues some pregnant women and air travelers by choosing foods carefully, avoiding carbonated drinks, eating and drinking slowly, and not chewing gum (suck on hard candy instead) as the plane lifts off.

When you travel, it's a wise precaution to bring along a copy of your prenatal records and lab results. You should also identify a source of prenatal medical care at your destination. This could be a large maternity hospital or a family member's or friend's obstetrician.

Working

Most pregnant women can work as long as they'd like. A 1978 amendment to Title VII of the 1964 Civil Rights Act prohibits job discrimination based on pregnancy, childbirth, or related medical conditions. In other words, you shouldn't be treated differently—demoted, denied advancement, or forced to resign—just because you're expecting a baby.

But if your pregnancy is considered high-risk (see Chapter 6), you may need to leave your job before you planned. Ask your prenatal caregiver for individual guidelines. You may, for example, be advised to stop working early or cut back on work time if you're pregnant with more than one baby, or if your history includes any of these problems:

▲ stillbirths, premature births, or second trimester miscarriages;
▲ an incompetent cervix or cerclage (a stitch to keep your cervix closed during pregnancy);

▲ heart, lung, blood, or kidney disease;

▲ severe diabetes;

▲ bleeding during pregnancy; or

▲ uterine malformations that threaten premature birth.

Legally, employers must treat these and other pregnancy-related conditions the same way they treat other temporary illnesses or disabilities. Ask your employer whether you're entitled to disability payments until you can return to work. Or you may qualify for unemployment or temporary disability payments from your state. Check with your state employment office, and don't be intimidated by the forms; your caregiver has probably filled them out many times.

Maybe you have a problem not with your pregnancy but with the type of job you hold. Before you get pregnant, or at your first appointment, talk to your caregiver about where you work and what your job involves. For example, if you regularly lift heavy objects, strain, climb stairs, or stand still for long periods, ask your caregiver whether you'll need to cut back your hours and how long you should continue working. If your job includes exposure to other dangers (see page 4), you may need to change how you work.

Do you work at a computer? Video display terminals (VDTs) don't pose risks to unborn babies (see page 4). But sitting at a keyboard, looking at a screen, may cause neck, back, wrist, hand, and shoulder pain, as well as eyestrain and psychological stress. If you work at a desk job during pregnancy—

▲ Sit in a chair that supports your lower back.

▲ Elevate your feet on a footstool or low desk drawer to minimize back pain.

▲ Adjust the height of your desk and chair to prevent discomfort in your neck, back, and arms.

▲ Set your computer screen at or just below eye level to reduce neck and back strain.

▲ Don't sit still for hours; take a short exercise break every hour or two.

▲ Between breaks, keep your muscles relaxed and your circulation going by shrugging and dropping your shoulders, slowly rolling your head, and rotating your feet.

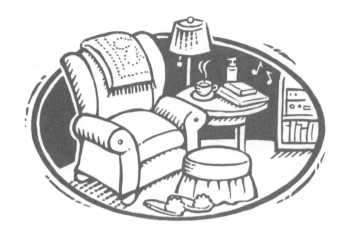

CHAPTER 5

Easing Pregnancy Aches and Pains

Some women sail through nine months of pregnancy with barely a twinge. But most women experience at least a few of the symptoms listed on page 81.

Keep in mind that most of these annoyances are normal and temporary, and that you can take simple steps to prevent or relieve quite a few. Be sure to discuss with your prenatal caregiver any symptoms that fail to respond to preventive measures or nonmedical treatments. To make it easier for you to find the information you need, pregnancy aches and pains are discussed here in alphabetical order.

ABDOMINAL, GROIN, OR RIB PAIN

After mid-pregnancy, the ligaments supporting your uterus may contract painfully when you sneeze, cough, laugh, or move too quickly. Pulling the round ligaments in the groin causes a sharp, shooting groin pain; pulling the ligaments attached to the ovaries causes a one-sided tug or twinge. An achy pain by the rib muscles is also common; so is a tugging sensation around your navel as your abdomen stretches.

Pregnancy Symptoms

Abdominal, groin, or rib pain
Allergies
Backache
Breast changes
Breathlessness
Constipation
Contractions
Dizziness or fainting
Emotional shifts
Fatigue
Food aversions
Food (and non-food) cravings
Gas
Gum bleeding
Headaches
Heart pounding
Heartburn or indigestion
Hemorrhoids
Hip, buttock, and thigh pain
Incontinence

Insomnia
Itchy abdomen
Leg cramps
Nausea ("morning sickness")
Nosebleeds
Numb fingers
Pelvic pain
Rashes
Rib discomfort
Salivation
Sciatica
Skin color changes
Stretch marks
Swelling of feet, ankles, or genital area
Urinary frequency
Urinary tract infections
Vaginal discharge, irritation, or infection
Varicose veins
Vision changes and eye irritation

What to do:

▲ Move slowly, allowing your ligaments to stretch slowly.
▲ If you can predict a sneeze or cough, pull up your legs to reduce pull on the ligaments.
▲ Gently massaging the painful area may relieve a cramp.
▲ Call your caregiver if pain lasts longer than a minute or two.

ALLERGIES

About one in seven pregnant women suffers chronic or seasonal allergies (see also Asthma, page 102). Some lucky women find that these allergies become less noticeable during pregnancy. Others find that their symptoms stay the same or get worse. Typical allergy symptoms—stuffed or runny nose, hives, rashes, watering eyes, sneezing, and coughing—pose no risk to pregnancy, but they may require medical attention if they keep you from eating or sleeping.

What to do:

- ▲ Avoid your worst offenders. For example, have your partner do the dusting and vacuuming; eliminate dust catchers such as drapes, blinds, and rugs; get rid of down quilts and feather pillows; stay away from foods that give you trouble; use an air conditioner or air filter to limit airborne allergens; stay inside in the mornings and on sunny, windy days; keep pets out of your bedroom; and avoid the basement if you're allergic to molds.
- ▲ Tell smokers you do mind if they smoke around you, and ask your employer to establish a smoke-free workplace. Smoke exacerbates other allergies and can trigger asthma.
- ▲ Use saline nose drops or spray to clear your nose.
- ▲ If coughing or sneezing makes you leak urine (see page 90), remember to do Kegel exercises (see page 63).
- ▲ Forego taking allergy medications during the first trimester, and ask your caregiver which ones you might safely use afterward. If you need an antihistamine, chlorpheniramine (in Chlor-Trimetron and other products) is probably a good choice. Decongestants such as oxymetazoline (in Afrin, Dristan, and other products) are best taken in the form of nasal sprays and drops; anti-allergy nasal sprays with cromolyn sodium (Intal and other products) are also considered safe during pregnancy.

BACKACHE

Pregnancy hormones loosen your joints and soften your muscles. As your pregnancy progresses, increasing weight pulls your spine forward. This may cause lower back strain. Upper back pain may result from heavier breasts pulling your shoulders forward.

What to do:

- ▲ Practice good posture, tucking your buttocks in and pulling your shoulders back (see page 61).
- ▲ Avoid standing still for prolonged periods. When standing, lift one foot onto a stool or other support.

- ▲ When lifting objects, bend from your knees, not your back (see page 62).
- ▲ Wear supportive, low-heeled shoes.
- ▲ When sitting, cushion your lower back with a pillow, and use a foot rest.
- ▲ Do pelvic-tilt exercises (see page 65).
- ▲ Use a heating pad or hot water bottle.
- ▲ Get a back rub.
- ▲ For upper back pain, try rolling your head in slow circles, or your shoulders forward and backward, and wear a supportive bra.

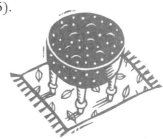

BREAST CHANGES

Your breasts will probably get heavier as your milk glands enlarge and fatty tissue increases in preparation for nursing. Your breasts may also become more sensitive. Near the end of pregnancy, your nipples may leak colostrum, a yellow substance that precedes breast milk.

What to do:

- ▲ Wear a supportive bra in your new size; you may need to purchase a maternity or nursing bra.
- ▲ If it helps, wear a comfortable bra at night.
- ▲ Practice good posture, pulling your shoulders back.
- ▲ If you leak colostrum, use cotton or gauze pads to absorb the fluid.
- ▲ Wash your nipples with plain water; soap can dry or irritate them.

BREATHLESSNESS

You may feel short of breath as your growing baby pushes your abdominal organs toward your chest, crowding your diaphragm.

What to do:

- ▲ Try to take slow, complete breaths.
- ▲ Hold your arms over your head and stretch.
- ▲ Experiment with different sleeping positions.
- ▲ Rest after any exercise.
- ▲ Avoid traveling to high-altitude areas in late pregnancy.

CONSTIPATION

Pregnancy hormones slow digestion, and the growing uterus puts pressure on the intestines. Those changes cause constipation in some pregnant women. Iron or vitamin supplements can also contribute to the problem.

What to do:

- ▲ Drink at least eight cups of fluid each day; warm liquids may be especially helpful.
- ▲ Eat plenty of high-fiber foods, including fresh fruits and vegetables, whole grains, and dried fruits such as prunes and figs.
- ▲ Get regular exercise, such as brisk walking, cycling, or swimming.
- ▲ Eliminate as soon as you feel the urge to do so, whenever possible.
- ▲ Avoid excessive iron supplementation.
- ▲ Unless your caregiver recommends them, avoid enemas and laxatives; mineral oil, for example, drives essential fat-soluble vitamins out of the body.
- ▲ Ask your caregiver if you should use a bulk-forming substance such as Metamucil or Citrucel or a gentle laxative such as Senokot or milk of magnesia.

CONTRACTIONS

After mid-pregnancy, Braxton-Hicks contractions (intermittent tightenings of the uterus) promote uterine circulation, prepare your uterus for labor, and eventually press the baby lower into your pelvis. These contractions commonly increase with exercise, and they are more frequent and noticeable during second and subsequent pregnancies.

What to do:

- ▲ If your contractions cause you discomfort, consciously relax the rest of your body.
- ▲ Drink a couple of glasses of water; contractions can be caused by dehydration.
- ▲ Use Braxton-Hicks contractions to practice your prepared childbirth techniques.
- ▲ Call your caregiver if you have more than four contractions per hour (one every 15 minutes) or if they continue for longer than one hour (see page 164).

Dizziness or Fainting

As your circulatory system pumps more blood to your uterus and fetus, at times it may rob blood from your brain. The result can be dizziness or fainting. Your increased blood volume may also make it hard to stay in one position for long or to adjust to quick position changes. Dehydration, overheating, or low blood sugar can make you feel dizzy, too.

What to do:

▲ Avoid standing or sitting still for long periods.

▲ Change slowly from one position to another.

▲ Avoid lying flat on your back after the fourth month of pregnancy; this position compresses your blood vessels and lowers blood pressure.

▲ Keep your shower or bath temperature at 100 degrees or lower (see page 72).

▲ Sleep on your side, or, if you prefer to lie on your back, use pillows to prop your back or one hip.

▲ If you feel faint, lie on your side until the feeling passes. Or sit or squat with your head between your knees, if you can't lie down.

▲ Be sure you have had enough fluids and small, frequent, not-too-sugary snacks.

Emotional Shifts

During pregnancy, high and fluctuating hormone levels may mimic PMS; fatigue and anxiety can also affect your mood. Some women feel unusually calm and contented during pregnancy.

What to do:

▲ Eat well, exercise, and get enough rest.

▲ Talk to your partner, friends, and family about your concerns.

▲ To ease anxiety about childbirth and the postpartum period, take classes to prepare yourself.

▲ Meet and talk to other expectant women who share your feelings.

▲ Pamper yourself with "feel good" treats, such as relaxation exercises (see page 67), listening to music, or catnaps.

FATIGUE

The hormonal changes of early pregnancy make most women tired; so does carrying around 25 to 30 pounds of extra weight toward the end of pregnancy. Anemia or low blood sugar could also cause fatigue.

What to do:

- ▲ Rest or catnap frequently during the day.
- ▲ Exercise regularly to give yourself an energy boost.
- ▲ Get help with household chores.
- ▲ Eat small, frequent meals to maintain your blood sugar.
- ▲ When you have extra energy, prepare nutritious snacks for later (see page 46).
- ▲ Be sure your caregiver routinely checks you for anemia. You may need to boost your intake of iron-rich foods or take an iron supplement (see page 53).
- ▲ Alert your caregiver if your fatigue is disabling. You could be suffering from an infection such as mononucleosis or a condition such as hypothyroidism.
- ▲ Be realistic: If you're a compulsive overachiever, learn to pace yourself and ask for help.

FOOD AVERSIONS

If you can't stand the smell or taste of foods you used to love, such as coffee or pizza, hormonal changes are probably responsible. Be patient. Food aversions usually fade somewhat after the first trimester.

What to do:

- ▲ Get someone else to cook.
- ▲ Substitute other foods that meet your nutritional needs.
- ▲ Don't worry if your diet is rather monotonous in the first trimester.
- ▲ Avoid bad smells. You may be able to eat your dinner if you don't have to smell it first.

FOOD (AND NON-FOOD) CRAVINGS

You may crave certain foods because you need extra nutrients or calories, or because of hormonal changes. Feel free to indulge your cravings so long as you keep eating nutritiously.

You may also feel tempted to consume a nonfood substance such as clay, starch, or dirt. Perhaps you think that eating this substance will ease birth. It won't. In fact, the substance may contain toxins or decrease your appetite for nutritious food.

What to do:

- ▲ Eat well (see Chapter 4).
- ▲ Have a light, high-protein snack before bedtime to stave off middle-of-the-night munchies.
- ▲ Avoid eating nonfood substances. If nonfood cravings continue or you can't tolerate a balanced diet, talk to your caregiver. You might request a referral to a registered dietitian.

GAS

In late pregnancy your growing uterus presses on your intestines, and pregnancy hormones slow your digestive system. This may make you feel gassy.

What to do:

- ▲ Avoid foods that make gas worse (the usual suspects are beans, peas, peanuts, cabbage and related vegetables, dried fruits, and wheat germ and bran).
- ▲ If milk disagrees with you, choose other calcium-rich foods that don't give you gas (see page 49).
- ▲ Sip, don't gulp, fluids.
- ▲ Avoid using a straw.
- ▲ Avoid chewing gum.
- ▲ Eat slowly, and take a walk after your meal.
- ▲ Avoid constipation (see page 84).

GUM BLEEDING

Increased blood volume and hormonal changes make your gums more sensitive. They may bleed easily when you brush or floss. To keep these changes from leading to infection, good dental care is important.

What to do:

- ▲ See your dentist before getting pregnant or early in pregnancy.

▲ Have your teeth and gums professionally cleaned every
six months; make sure your dentist knows that you are
pregnant.

▲ Brush your teeth with a soft-bristle toothbrush after
every meal, and floss twice a day.

▲ Eat two foods high in vitamin C every day (see page 51).

HEADACHES

The hormonal and circulatory changes of pregnancy can cause
headaches. They are most common at 9 to 10 weeks, when hormones peak, and during rapid blood volume increases at 16 to 18
weeks and 26 to 28 weeks. Headaches can also arise from stress,
from sinus problems, or from caffeine withdrawal.

What to do:

▲ Try relaxation exercises (see page 67).

▲ Apply a warm, moist towel to your eyes and forehead.

▲ Reduce caffeine intake gradually.

▲ Consult your caregiver before taking any painkiller.

▲ For sinus headaches, drink plenty of fluids, use a humidifier to loosen mucus, and make sure your glasses fit
right; glasses that pinch the bridge of the nose can boost
sinus pain.

▲ Report a severe, persistent headache to your caregiver;
it could be a sign of preeclampsia (see page 115).

HEART POUNDING

An occasional rapid heartbeat is normal as your circulatory system adapts to an increasing blood volume.

What to do:

▲ Try relaxation exercises (see page 67).

▲ Slow down your breathing.

▲ Call your caregiver if heart pounding is accompanied by
fainting, chest pain, or severe shortness of breath.

HEARTBURN OR INDIGESTION

The hormonal changes of pregnancy slow your digestion and
relax the muscles of your esophagus, letting stomach acids back
up.

What to do:

- ▲ Eat several small meals and snacks each day instead of three large ones.
- ▲ Eat slowly.
- ▲ Avoid fatty and gas-producing foods (see page 87).
- ▲ Don't eat just before bedtime.
- ▲ Stay upright after eating.
- ▲ Try chewing gum, if gas isn't a problem for you.
- ▲ Consult your prenatal caregiver before taking antacids.

HEMORRHOIDS

Varicose veins of the rectum, hemorrhoids are common in pregnancy, when an increased blood volume dilates the veins and pressure from the growing uterus slows the return of blood to the heart. Straining while eliminating makes hemorrhoids worse.

What to do:

- ▲ Do Kegel exercises daily (see page 63) to encourage good circulation in your pelvic area.
- ▲ Avoid constipation (see page 84).
- ▲ Support your feet on a small footstool when using the toilet.
- ▲ Keep from straining while eliminating by breathing out as you push.
- ▲ Make compresses by soaking cotton balls in cold witch hazel; apply them while lying on your side.
- ▲ If witch hazel doesn't help, ask your caregiver to recommend a stool softener containing docusate (Surfak, Dialose, and Calace, for example) or a hemorrhoidal cream or ointment to lubricate your rectum.

HIP, BUTTOCK, AND THIGH PAIN

In late pregnancy, hormones loosen your joints. This can make it painful to support the extra weight of your baby.

What to do:

- ▲ Let someone else carry heavy items.
- ▲ Choose low-impact aerobic exercise, such as walking or swimming, over exercises such as jogging that increase strain on your hips and legs.

INCONTINENCE

Because your growing uterus puts extra stress on your pelvic floor muscles and presses against your bladder, you may leak urine at times. Certain foods can contribute to this problem.

What to do:

▲ Do at least 80 Kegels a day (see page 63).

▲ Tighten your pelvic floor muscles before you climb stairs, change positions, lift, laugh, cough, or sneeze.

▲ Choose low-impact aerobic exercise, such as walking or swimming, over high-impact exercise, such as jogging.

▲ Keep drinking eight cups of liquid a day; restricting fluids worsens the problem.

▲ Avoid constipation (see page 84).

▲ One at a time, try eliminating possible bladder irritants from your diet: caffeine, highly acidic fruits such as grapefruit, tomatoes, and sugar.

▲ Avoid allergens if you're sneezing a lot (see page 82).

▲ Consult your caregiver if these measures fail to help.

INSOMNIA

Discomfort from your extra weight and bulk, the need to urinate frequently, hunger, nightmares, or caffeine too close to bedtime may keep you awake.

What to do:

▲ Treat yourself to extra pillows and experiment with them until you find a comfortable sleeping position.

▲ Get some regular daily exercise, but avoid exercising within two hours of bedtime.

▲ Establish and stick to a regular bedtime routine.

▲ Use relaxation techniques to help you drift off to sleep (see pages 67 to 71).

▲ Take a warm bath or shower before going to bed.

▲ Have a light snack, including a glass of milk, near bedtime.

▲ Reduce or eliminate caffeine in your diet, especially in the afternoon and evening.

ITCHY ABDOMEN

This is caused by the tight stretching of skin across your abdomen.

What to do:

- ▲ Limit scratching, which only makes itching worse.
- ▲ Use lotion or cream to lubricate the area.
- ▲ Try an anti-itching agent, such as calamine lotion.
- ▲ Avoid electric blankets, which can dry your skin.

LEG CRAMPS

By slowing circulation in your legs, pressure from your growing uterus may cause leg cramps. A dietary imbalance between calcium and phosphorus can also trigger muscle cramps.

What to do:

- ▲ Limit carbonated beverages, lunch meats, and other processed foods containing phosphorus, which interferes with calcium absorption.
- ▲ Drink 4 cups of milk a day, but no more, because the phosphorus in milk could also cause cramps. If you can't tolerate milk, substitute other calcium-rich foods (see page 49), or ask your caregiver to recommend a calcium supplement.
- ▲ Avoid pointing your toes, which could trigger a cramp.
- ▲ If you get a calf cramp, stand up, or stretch out of it by pushing your heel down while pointing your toe up toward your face. Or have your partner press down on your knee with one hand and with the other push up on the ball of your foot.

NAUSEA ("MORNING SICKNESS")

Hormonal changes are usually to blame. Though nausea in pregnancy is called morning sickness, it can occur at any time of day. Nausea sometimes lasts well beyond the first trimester.

What to do:

- ▲ Eat a high-protein snack before bedtime.
- ▲ Leave crackers, toast, or dry unsweetened cereal by your bedside to eat first thing in the morning.
- ▲ Have a snack of toast or crackers whenever you feel queasy.

- ▲ Eat small, frequent meals each day instead of three large ones.
- ▲ Because you may be more apt to keep down liquids drunk between meals, try postponing your drink for an hour or so after you eat.
- ▲ Increase your intake of foods rich in vitamin B₆—whole grains, nuts, seeds, peanuts, and corn—or ask your caregiver about taking a supplement.
- ▲ Consider acupuncture, which the National Institutes of Health recently recognized as an effective treatment for this problem, or try acupressure (see illustration). Wristbands such as Sea Bands, sold in drugstores for seasickness, can also be helpful.

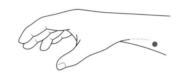

Press hard on this point with the opposite thumb for a minute or two.

- ▲ With your caregiver's okay, take ginger supplements, available at health food stores. You might also try ginger tea or candied ginger.
- ▲ Since undernourishment and dehydration could pose risks for you and your baby, call your prenatal caregiver if vomiting persists. Prescription medication or IV fluids may be needed.

NOSEBLEEDS
Increased blood volume and hormonal changes that dry your nasal passages can cause your nose to bleed.

What to do:

- ▲ To moisten the air in your house, use a humidifier. Be sure to clean it regularly.
- ▲ With an eye dropper, insert a few drops of warm water into your nose several times a day.
- ▲ Be gentle when you blow your nose.
- ▲ If you get a nosebleed, pinch your nostrils shut tightly for ten minutes, or apply an ice pack to the bridge of your nose to stop the bleeding.
- ▲ Ask your prenatal caregiver before using antihistamines for a stuffy nose.
- ▲ Avoid medications that contain aspirin or ibuprofen.

NUMB FINGERS

The cause could be carpal tunnel syndrome, in which extra body fluid causes swelling in the wrist's carpal tunnel. Through this narrow opening nerves and blood vessels pass to the hand; the swelling compresses the median nerve that supplies the thumb and next three fingers.

What to do:

- ▲ Avoid sleeping on your hands or with bent wrists.
- ▲ Use pillows to prop your head and shoulders while sleeping.
- ▲ Try wearing a wrist splint, available at drugstores.
- ▲ Ask your prenatal caregiver about taking extra vitamin B_6; it works as a diuretic and also improves nerve function.
- ▲ Call your caregiver if the swelling is sudden or occurs in your face as well as your fingers. Severe swelling may signal preeclampsia (see page 115).

PELVIC PAIN

As hormones relax your pelvic joints and circulation changes cause blood to pool in your pelvis, it may ache.

What to do:

- ▲ Avoid constipation (see page 84).
- ▲ Do Kegel exercises (page 63) daily to improve pelvic circulation.
- ▲ Rest with pillows under your hips to promote the return of blood to your heart.
- ▲ Try an ice pack between your legs to numb the pelvic area.
- ▲ Avoid heat, which encourages blood flow to the area.

RASHES

You may get a rash called prickly heat if part of your body rubs against another part—your breasts against your chest, for example, or your lower abdomen against your groin. A different condition, called **PUPP** (pruritic urticarial papules and plaques of pregnancy) may appear as itchy, reddish, raised areas first on your belly and then on your limbs. PUPP, which can run in families, rarely reappears after a woman's first pregnancy. This itchy condition doesn't threaten the baby.

What to do:

- ▲ Prevent or treat prickly heat by drying yourself thoroughly and applying talcum powder after bathing.
- ▲ Relieve itching by soaking in a warm bath to which you have added baking soda or oatmeal.
- ▲ Ask your caregiver to recommend oral medication or an anti-itching product, such as calamine lotion.

RIB DISCOMFORT

Because the growing uterus forces your rib cage to stay expanded, it may sometimes feel sore.

What to do:

- ▲ Try to breathe slowly.
- ▲ Stretch with your arms over your head.
- ▲ Practice good posture (see page 61).

SALIVATION

Pregnancy causes your salivary glands to step up production.

What to do:

- ▲ Chew gum, if it helps.
- ▲ Eat several small meals each day instead of three large ones.

SCIATICA

As your lower back curves to accommodate your growing belly, the sciatic nerve that runs from your lower back through your pelvis and upper leg may get pinched.

What to do:

- ▲ Avoid heavy lifting.
- ▲ Always lift with bent legs.
- ▲ Try the standing pelvic tilt (see page 67).
- ▲ When standing, elevate one foot on a book or low stool.

SKIN COLOR CHANGES

Hormonal changes darken your freckles, the areolas around your nipples, and the line down the center of your abdomen (*linea nigra*). Hormones can also cause mask-like spots or patches (*chloasma*) to appear on your face.

What to do:

- ▲ Experiment with makeup to camouflage facial coloring changes.
- ▲ Avoid sunlight: Use a wide-brimmed hat and apply a sun block with an SPF (sun protection factor) of 15 or higher.
- ▲ Keep in mind that the dark coloration will probably fade after the birth, although it may not completely disappear.

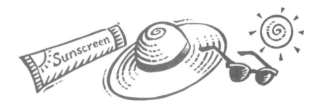

STRETCH MARKS

Your rapid increase in size and weight during pregnancy makes your skin stretch. This stretching may cause the tearing of collagen fibers in the skin of your lower abdomen, breasts, buttocks, or thighs.

What to do:

- ▲ Exercise to strengthen the muscles that support the skin in these areas. Try the pelvic tilt (page 66), walking, swimming, or stationary cycling.
- ▲ Wear a supportive, well-fitting bra.
- ▲ Use cream or lotion to reduce dryness and itching.
- ▲ Keep eating sensibly; though excessive weight gain can result in unnecessary stretch marks, over-restricting your weight gain won't prevent them.
- ▲ Keep in mind that stretch marks fade after pregnancy.

SWELLING OF FEET, ANKLES, OR GENITAL AREA

Some swelling is normal in late pregnancy, when your growing uterus compresses the blood vessels that return blood from the lower part of your body. Swelling in your face and hands, however, can mean preeclampsia (see page 115), and demands an immediate call to your caregiver.

What to do:

- ▲ Avoid standing or sitting still for long periods.
- ▲ Several times a week, walk, swim, or ride a stationary bike to promote circulation in your legs.
- ▲ Avoid crossing your legs while sitting.
- ▲ Two or three times a day, lie down for 15 to 20 minutes. Use pillows to prop your legs higher than your heart, or lie on your side.
- ▲ Use a rocking chair to give the muscles in your feet and legs a mini-workout.
- ▲ Avoid tight socks and pants that might impair your circulation.
- ▲ Because the major blood vessel that drains your lower body lies just right of your mid-spine, lie on your left side to sleep; don't lie flat on your back.
- ▲ Keep drinking plenty of fluids; restricting fluids can worsen swelling.
- ▲ Maternity support hose can help promote the circulation that eases swelling, but avoid calf and thigh-high stockings, which would compress your blood vessels.

URINARY FREQUENCY

Early and late in pregnancy, the pressure of the enlarging uterus presses on the bladder, causing a frequent urge to urinate. Toward the end of pregnancy, increased blood volume contributes to the problem.

What to do:

- ▲ Scout out bathrooms wherever you travel.
- ▲ Empty your bladder completely each time you urinate.
- ▲ Avoid restricting fluids; your kidneys need plenty of water to keep functioning.
- ▲ Call your caregiver if you feel burning or stinging when you urinate; you may have a urinary tract infection.

URINARY TRACT INFECTIONS

Frequent urination boosts the risk for these infections.

What to do:

▲ Wear cotton panties.

▲ Avoid clothing that is tight in the crotch.

▲ Avoid using feminine hygiene sprays, perfumed bubble bath, or douches. Douching not only increases the risk of urinary tract infections but can spread a vaginal infection into the uterus or introduce an air bubble into your blood system.

▲ Empty your bladder completely after intercourse and every time you urinate.

▲ Wipe yourself from front to back after using the toilet.

▲ Drink 8 cups of water each day.

▲ Drink cranberry juice and eat citrus fruits to acidify your urine and make urinary tract infections less likely.

▲ If you experience one or more symptoms of a urinary tract infection—a burning sensation while urinating, blood in the urine, or a frequent, urgent need to urinate—call your caregiver immediately.

VAGINAL DISCHARGE, IRRITATION, OR INFECTION

During pregnancy, blood circulation and hormonal changes increase vaginal secretions and render them less acidic. This may set the stage for vaginal irritation or infection. A **yeast infection** causes a cheesy, white vaginal discharge, a burning sensation, and itching. You can buy an over-the-counter yeast medication, but consult your caregiver to confirm the diagnosis first. Another type of organism can cause an infection called **trichomoniasis.** Symptoms include a gray or green foul-smelling discharge, along with itching and burning. If your caregiver diagnoses "trich," you will need a prescription medication to treat it. To avoid reinfection, your partner should also be treated.

What to do:

▲ Follow the instructions on this page for preventing urinary tract infections. In particular, wear cotton panties, and avoid vaginal sprays and douches.

▲ Use mini-pads or pantiliners sparingly when you need to protect your clothing. Cotton panties keep the area dryer.

▲ If you have a vaginal infection, try relieving the discomfort with frequent warm baths.

▲ Alert your caregiver if your vaginal discharge itches, smells bad, or stings.

▲ Contact your caregiver if the discharge is blood-tinged, which could indicate a miscarriage or ectopic pregnancy. Watery discharge could also be a sign of labor (see page 169).

VARICOSE VEINS

Increased blood volume and the pressure of the expanding uterus slow circulation and dilate veins in the legs.

What to do:

▲ Avoid standing still for prolonged periods.

▲ Don't sit cross-legged.

▲ Rest several times a day with your feet up.

▲ Wear maternity support stockings. If your varicose veins are painful, ask your caregiver about prescription-strength surgical hose.

VISION CHANGES AND EYE IRRITATION

Pregnancy hormones can contribute to temporary vision changes; increased circulation may make wearing contact lenses uncomfortable or result in minor prescription changes. In addition, your eyes may feel dry or sensitive.

What to do:

▲ To soothe dry eyes, use an over-the-counter "artificial tears" product.

▲ If your contacts bother you, temporarily switch to glasses or disposable soft contacts.

▲ If possible, delay getting a new prescription for glasses or contact lenses until after the birth.

▲ If you do get a new prescription for glasses during pregnancy, save your old lenses; you may be able to use them again after the birth.

▲ Promptly report to your prenatal caregiver any sudden visual changes. Blurring, double vision, or blind spots can occasionally result from high blood pressure or signal preeclampsia (see page 115).

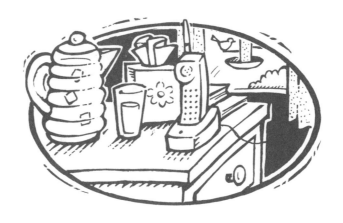

CHAPTER 6

Difficult Pregnancies

Until recently in this country, and to this day in certain parts of the world, pregnancy has been risky and life-threatening. Today most women in developed countries enjoy good nutrition, a safe water supply, and, when medical problems or pregnancy complications arise, state-of-the-art medical care.

But even under the best of circumstances, pregnancy can be a challenge. And some pregnancies definitely pose more problems than others. Some pregnancies are risky from the beginning, while others start smoothly, only to develop difficulties as time passes.

This chapter covers some of the conditions that can complicate an expectant mother's life. Read straight through, this chapter could make pregnancy sound like a minefield. To avoid becoming unnecessarily frightened, read only the parts that apply to you or that you have questions about. Keep in mind that most pregnancies sail along without a ripple. Then bring your concerns and questions to your caregiver, and breathe a little easier. Remember that most pregnancies, even the high-risk ones, end happily.

———·❤·———

Are You at Risk?

Experts don't all agree on what constitutes a high-risk pregnancy. If your prenatal caregiver tells you your pregnancy is high-risk, make sure you understand why. Then ask for the information and support you need to take good care of yourself and your baby.

The risks that follow include pre-existing maternal conditions, pregnancy-related illnesses, and fetal characteristics. They're discussed in alphabetical order to make it easier for you to find the topics you need.

Age

At any age, you have an excellent chance to deliver a healthy baby. Of course, your general good health boosts the odds for a safe delivery. Also crucial are getting prenatal care and looking after yourself—eating well, exercising, and avoiding harmful habits like smoking, drinking, and using recreational drugs. But if you are under nineteen or in your late thirties or older, you do run some extra risks.

TEEN MOTHERS   Women in their twenties can usually get pregnant quickly, are less likely than older or younger mothers to have a miscarriage or cesarean delivery, and run the lowest risk of bearing a baby with chromosomal problems. Still, giving birth in your teens can be as risky as having a baby when you are over 35. For example, teenagers experience higher rates of preeclampsia than do women in their twenties and early thirties. Teen mothers are also more likely to deliver early.

Most of the problems of teen pregnancy stem from elements of lifestyle, such as poor diet, poverty, smoking, or drug use, and from failure to get prenatal care. But even when teens eat well and get prenatal care, they still experience higher rates of placental problems and cesarean births than do women in their twenties and early thirties. The younger the teen, the higher the risk.

Experts believe that physical immaturity contributes to the extra risks young mothers face. For example, cesareans may be more common among teens because some of them have not yet reached full body stature and because their bodies may not make enough relaxin. This hormone relaxes the pelvic ligaments, allowing the pelvic bones to expand for the birth.

On the bright side, teen parents often have more physical energy for labor and infant care. In addition, their younger, more active parents can often pitch in to help with housekeeping and child-care tasks.

MOTHERS OVER 35   If you're having your first child after your thirtieth birthday, you have plenty of company. In 1975 only 5 percent of first births occurred to women 30 years of age and older. By 2002, one in four first births were to the over-30 set. Today many women are marrying later and completing their education or launching a career before beginning their families.

The good news is that a healthy pregnant woman in her early thirties faces about the same risks as a woman in her twenties. But your chance for problems does rise slowly along with your age. First of all, fertility declines, so you may find it harder to get pregnant. When you do get pregnant, you may get more babies than you bargained for: The incidence of multiple births climbs for mothers over 35 and peaks between 45 and 54.

Women in their late thirties and older also have higher rates of conditions such as diabetes and hypertension, which can threaten pregnancy. In addition, older women are more likely to be obese, which raises the risk of gestational diabetes, preeclampsia, and cesarean delivery.

Even in healthy mothers, the risk of giving birth to a baby with chromosomal abnormalities rises with age (see page 106). Because most miscarriages are of abnormal fetuses, older women experience a higher rate of miscarriage. Older mothers also have a higher chance of experiencing—

- ▲ pregnancy-induced hypertension (see page 106);
- ▲ placental problems such as placenta previa, in which the placenta blocks the cervix, and placental abruption, in which the placenta detaches from the uterine wall (see page 143);
- ▲ breech presentation (see page 103); and
- ▲ stillbirth.

But being older has advantages, too. Women over 35 are usually well prepared for pregnancy. They more often avoid toxins, get good prenatal care, maintain a healthy diet, and exercise. Because women over 35 are typically counseled about the availability of genetic testing, in some areas they deliver babies with chromosomal abnormalities at lower rates than do their younger counterparts.

Talk to your prenatal caregiver about whether your age alone puts you at risk and, if so, in what ways your pregnancy may be handled differently because of this. Ask about any aspect of your care you don't understand. Take good care of yourself and your baby during pregnancy, and have confidence in your body's wisdom. Remember that the vast majority of babies are born healthy no matter how old their mothers are.

Asthma

One to four out of 100 pregnant women have asthma. Most pregnant women with this respiratory condition notice no change in their symptoms, and some even enjoy an improvement. But about one-third of asthmatic pregnant women—typically women with severe cases—find that their symptoms temporarily worsen.

Left uncontrolled, asthma can reduce the amount of oxygen that reaches a baby and this lack of oxygen can trigger premature delivery or low birth weight. Uncontrolled asthma also boosts the mother's risk for preeclampsia (see page 115). The good news is that controlled asthma should not threaten the baby's health, and that most asthma medications pose little risk in pregnancy.

To keep asthma from affecting your pregnancy, consult the doctor who treats the condition before pregnancy or as soon as you find out you're pregnant. During pregnancy, take these steps to prevent asthmatic episodes or decrease their impact:

▲ Avoid smoking or inhaling secondhand smoke.

▲ Avoid exposure to colds and other respiratory infections.

▲ If you catch a bug, ask your doctor which medications you should take to ward off an asthma attack.

▲ Get a flu shot in the fall.

▲ Ask your doctor about using a bronchodilator immediately before exercising.

▲ If you have an asthma attack, treat it promptly with the medication your doctor has prescribed, and notify your doctor if your symptoms worsen.

Autoimmune Disease

These illnesses occur when the body, mistaking its own tissue for an intruder, produces antibodies that attack various parts of the body. Autoimmune diseases, which include **systemic lupus erythematosis, rheumatoid arthritis, chronic fatigue syndrome,** and **multiple sclerosis,** occur much more frequently in women than they do in men.

During pregnancy, a woman's normal immune response changes as her body curbs its tendency to reject foreign tissue. Perhaps for this reason, pregnancy may cause the symptoms of some autoimmune diseases—especially rheumatoid arthritis—to improve temporarily or even disappear. But some unlucky women find that their autoimmune disease flares up during pregnancy or soon afterwards. If possible, consult with your disease specialist before getting pregnant so you have a good idea of what to expect and to choose the safest medications.

Breech Presentation

At least 95 out of 100 babies settle into a head-down position in the weeks that precede birth. Fewer than one in 100 babies stay in a crosswise, or shoulder-first, position; these babies must be delivered by cesarean.

The breech presentation, in which the baby's bottom, feet, or legs come first, occurs only 3 to 4 percent of the time at full term but more often when a baby is premature or a twin. Because coming out bottom first poses a risk to your baby, ask your caregiver about trying to turn your baby to a head-down position before birth. Most babies assume their birth position by about 34 or 35 weeks. If your baby is still in the bottom first position at 36 weeks, encourage him to somersault by trying the **breech tilt position:**

▲ Lie on your back with your feet flat on the floor and your knees bent.

▲ Use cushions or an ironing board tilted with one end on a chair, to raise your hips about 12 inches higher than your head.

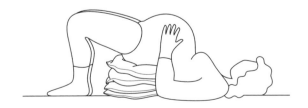

▲ Assume this position for 10 minutes three times each day when your baby is active.

In addition to, or instead of doing the breech tilt, some women try to lure their babies to turn around by playing music through earphones placed just above the pubic bone. The baby just might change position to hear the music better.

Another method of trying to turn a baby comes from Chinese medicine. An herb called mugwort is burned near the mother's little toe. Ask your caregiver whether there is any harm in trying this method.

If your baby remains breech at 37 to 38 weeks, your caregiver may try a medical procedure called **external version**—manually shifting the baby to a head-down position from the outside. Performed in the hospital with safeguards for the mother and baby, version succeeds about two-thirds of the time.

If your baby fails to turn or resumes a bottom-first position, your caregiver must decide whether it's safe to attempt a vaginal delivery. Since a safe vaginal delivery depends both on the baby's position and size and on your birth attendant's skill and experience, most babies who stay in the breech position enter the world by cesarean.

DES

Diethylstilbestrol, a synthetic estrogen, was used in the 1950s in a misguided attempt to prevent miscarriage. Women exposed to DES during their mothers' pregnancies may be unaffected or may have minor abnormalities in the uterus, fallopian tubes, or cervix. But some DES daughters have serious internal abnormalities, which raise their risks for miscarriage, ectopic pregnancy, and preterm labor.

If your mother took DES during her pregnancy with you, let your caregiver know as soon as possible.

Diabetes and Gestational Diabetes

About one pregnant woman in 100 has diabetes. A person with diabetes lacks or can't make use of insulin, the hormone that removes sugar from the blood and stores it in the body's cells. Chronic high levels of blood sugar can injure the mother's blood vessels, eyes, and kidneys. Uncontrolled diabetes in an expectant mother can result in miscarriage or stillbirth. Or it may cause serious problems, including abnormally high birth weight and associated complications; low blood sugar; jaundice; and breathing difficulties. To prevent these effects, women with diabetes may need to follow a diet designed to avoid high blood sugar, and some may need to inject themselves regularly with insulin. Specialized medical supervision beginning before pregnancy and careful self-monitoring can enable a diabetic woman to deliver a healthy baby.

Gestational diabetes is a form of diabetes that strikes 2 to 3 percent of women during the second or third trimester of pregnancy. The cause? Placental hormones that temporarily change the way insulin functions. Though blood sugar levels typically return to normal after delivery, women with gestational diabetes run a higher-than-average risk of developing the condition during future pregnancies and of developing adult-onset diabetes in later life. The most likely candidates to develop gestational diabetes are—

▲ pregnant women over 30,
▲ obese women,
▲ women with a family history of diabetes,
▲ women who have previously given birth to a baby weighing nine pounds or more, and
▲ women who have had an unexplained stillbirth.

Like uncontrolled regular diabetes, uncontrolled gestational diabetes puts mothers and babies at risk for serious problems. Because early detection and treatment can prevent these problems, a pregnant woman typically takes a **glucose test** to screen for gestational diabetes between 24 and 28 weeks (see page 37). If her blood sugar tests high, she takes the lengthier, more accurate **glucose tolerance test.** If the second test indicates gestational diabetes, her treatment may include a special diet (85 to 90 percent of women can control gestational diabetes through diet alone), supervised exercise, frequent checks of blood sugar levels, and, occasionally, insulin injections. If the baby appears to be growing too large, labor may be induced just before or at term. The caregiver usually orders nonstress tests (see page 40) and ultrasound scans (see page 34) to monitor the baby's growth pattern and the placental function.

Fetal Abnormalities

When prenatal testing reveals a serious birth defect, many parents choose to terminate the pregnancy. Others opt instead to plan for the birth of an ill or handicapped child. If you and your partner make this choice, your caregiver should respect your feelings, accept your decision, and provide or refer you to a hospital equipped to handle your newborn. During pregnancy, ask to meet with the pediatric expert who will care for your infant. In addition, seek out parents who have been through a similar experience. Your prenatal caregiver, a pediatrician, or a hospital social worker may be a good source for referrals.

Heart Disease

Pregnancy places extra demands on your circulatory system. Your blood volume expands by 50 percent, and, to supply the placenta and fetus, your heart pumps about one-third more blood with each beat. A healthy heart can meet these demands, but a woman with a heart problem such as rheumatic heart disease, a congenital defect, or artificial heart valves may find pregnancy a strain. Women with mild or moderate heart disease can usually safely undertake pregnancy under careful medical supervision.

If you have a heart problem, be sure to consult your cardiologist before becoming pregnant so that you can be sure of having a healthy baby and staying healthy yourself. You'll probably be advised to get extra rest every day, and you may have to spend much of your pregnancy on bed rest (see page 119). You're no more likely to need a cesarean than any other mother, but your doctor may want to deliver your baby with low outlet forceps (see page 141) or a vacuum extractor (see page 142) if it appears that the strain of pushing would otherwise cause problems for you.

Hypertension (High Blood Pressure)

Six to eight percent of pregnant women have hypertension—that is, blood pressure over 140 systolic (when the heart contracts) or 90 diastolic (when the heart rests). **Chronic hypertension** is high blood pressure diagnosed before pregnancy or before the twentieth week of pregnancy. **Pregnancy-induced hypertension (PIH)** is blood pressure that rises after the first 20 weeks of pregnancy or in the first 24 hours after delivery. Women with hypertension run a higher risk of developing preeclampsia or eclampsia (see page 115).

Hypertension can pose a serious risk to mother and child. It can decrease the baby's blood supply and interfere with his growth.

You're most likely to have high blood pressure or to develop it during pregnancy if you—

▲ smoke,
▲ are obese,
▲ have kidney disease,
▲ have a family history of hypertension,
▲ are over 35, or
▲ are pregnant with your first baby.

During pregnancy, treatment for hypertension includes—

▲ regular bed rest, preferably on the left side (see page 96) to promote good circulation;
▲ blood pressure monitoring;
▲ blood tests to detect possible blood and liver problems;
▲ nonstress tests (see page 40) and ultrasound scans (see page 34) to ensure that the placenta is functioning and the baby is moving normally;
▲ when necessary, medications to lower blood pressure; and
▲ induction of labor (see page 166) at term or sooner if hypertension endangers mother or baby.

Infections

A common cold or case of the flu shouldn't cause you any concern. But illnesses you may not have even noticed if you weren't pregnant can jeopardize your pregnancy or your baby. Some infections increase the rates of miscarriage and preterm delivery. A few infections can threaten birth defects or developmental problems for your baby, depending on when you catch the illness, whether you have antibodies to it, and whether you can be treated.

To safeguard your baby and yourself, try to avoid exposure to infectious diseases, and promptly report any of these symptoms of infection to your prenatal caregiver:

▲ fever of 100 degrees Fahrenheit or higher;
▲ severe or chronic headache or body aching all over;
▲ rash;
▲ lower respiratory symptoms;

▲ unusual vaginal discharge, or itching, burning, or stinging in the vagina;

▲ burning after urination.

BACTERIAL VAGINOSIS This common vaginal infection can boost your risk of pelvic inflammatory disease, miscarriage, and preterm labor. So call your caregiver promptly if you notice a cream-colored or grayish vaginal discharge that smells fishy, especially after a bath or sex. Treatment options for pregnant women include oral or topical metronidazole or oral clindamycin. If you experience recurrent episodes, your partner should also be treated, because bacterial vaginosis may be sexually transmitted. While either of you undergoes treatment, it's best to avoid intercourse or to use condoms.

CHICKEN POX Also called varicella, this common childhood disease leads to serious fetal malformations about 2 percent of the time when a mother becomes infected before the twentieth week of pregnancy.

When a mother catches chicken pox shortly before or shortly after delivery, her newborn can also become infected. Chicken pox is a serious disease in a newborn, but the infection can be prevented or limited by giving the baby an injection of chicken pox antibodies (varicella-zoster immune globulin, VZIG) right after birth. When given to a pregnant woman within 96 hours after her exposure to chicken pox, VZIG also helps prevent maternal complications such as pneumonia.

Fortunately, most women have immunity to chicken pox because they had the disease in childhood. A woman who lacks immunity can be vaccinated against the disease before pregnancy. Her children and partner should also get vaccinated if they're not immune already. But a woman should delay conception until at least three months after she and family members get their shots.

CHLAMYDIA Currently the most common sexually transmitted disease in the United States, chlamydia affects as many as one in eight pregnant women. This often symptomless infection can inflame the cervix or urethra. It also accounts for many cases of pelvic inflammatory disease, which can leave a woman infertile or cause a life-threatening ectopic pregnancy (see page 21).

A baby born to a mother with chlamydia risks eye infection or pneumonia.

Standard antibiotic treatments for chlamydia are considered unsafe during pregnancy, but the antibiotic erythromycin offers an effective alternative. Erythromycin ointment is also used after hospital delivery to prevent chlamydia-caused eye infections in newborns.

To prevent passing chlamydia back and forth between sexual partners, both should be treated whenever one has become infected. It's best to abstain from sexual intercourse until treatment is complete. Using condoms, however, may help reduce the risk of reinfection.

CYTOMEGALOVIRUS (CMV)   Fifty to 80 percent of adults have antibodies to this symptomless virus, for which there is no vaccine or treatment. Although your risk of catching CMV for the first time during pregnancy is only about 1 percent, you should take this risk seriously. One in ten exposed fetuses suffers serious birth defects or mental retardation, and one in five infected babies dies. Spread by infected bodily fluids, CMV can be prevented by hand-washing after contact with infants and young children.

FIFTH DISEASE   About 50 percent of women are immune to fifth disease, a common childhood illness that causes a cheek rash and is spread through the air. Most fetuses remain unaffected even if their mothers catch the virus, but some may develop anemia or heart failure. At highest risk of infection are mothers of young children and women who work with young children in day-care facilities, schools, medical clinics, and hospitals.

Talk to your caregiver if you've recently been exposed to fifth disease, because a new test can determine whether you have immunity. If you should become infected during pregnancy, you'll be carefully monitored for signs of fetal problems, which may be treatable in utero (see "Percutaneous Umbilical Blood Sampling" in Chapter 3).

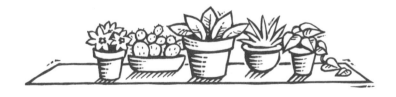

GROUP B STREPTOCOCCUS (GBS)   Unlike the Group A streptococcus that causes strep throat, this bacterial infection is carried in a woman's vagina or rectum. Ten to 30 percent of pregnant women carry GBS. Harmless to the mother, this infection can threaten a baby's life or cause cerebral palsy, sight or hearing loss, or mental retardation.

Researchers are working to develop a maternal vaccine to protect babies from GBS. For now, the U.S. Centers for Disease Control recommend testing all pregnant women at 34 to 36 weeks for vaginal or rectal infection with GBS and treating those with a positive culture with antibiotics during labor. Ask your prenatal caregiver about his or her practice. If you have had a GBS culture during pregnancy, make sure your hospital caregivers are aware of the results.

HEPATITIS B (HBV)   This liver virus, which is transmitted via blood and bodily fluids, strikes about 80,000 Americans each year. Hepatitis B usually causes nothing worse than mild flu-like symptoms in the teens and young adults who are its typical victims. But some babies become chronic hepatitis B carriers after catching the infection at birth. These babies run a much higher risk of later developing liver cancer or cirrhosis of the liver.

Most pregnant women are screened for HBV. Uninfected women who face the highest risk for the disease, including health-care workers and women with multiple sexual partners, should be vaccinated against HBV before or even during pregnancy.

Babies born to HBV carriers receive HBV vaccine and hepatitis B immune globulin at birth, a treatment that prevents 95 percent of them from becoming infected. Currently the American Academy of Pediatrics recommends that all hospital-born newborns be immunized against hepatitis B before being discharged.

HERPES   Closely related to the viruses that cause chicken pox, shingles, and mononucleosis, the herpes simplex virus causes cold sores and painful genital blisters. Although genital herpes is typically transmitted by genital intercourse, it can also result from oral-genital contact if one partner has a cold sore. There is no cure for genital herpes, but topical creams, baking soda baths, and cotton underpants offer relief from symptoms, and prescription medications can suppress or limit outbreaks.

If a mother has a flare-up of genital herpes at the time of delivery—especially if she has just contracted herpes—her infant risks contracting the virus in the birth canal. This rare event can cause blindness, brain damage, or death. If you have active herpes sores near your due date or experience the pain or itching that often precedes an outbreak, let your caregiver know. To safeguard your baby, you may need a cesarean delivery.

To keep from catching your partner's genital herpes during pregnancy, avoid sex when your partner's sores are active and use a condom at other times. In addition, avoid oral sex if you or your partner experiences a cold sore flare-up.

HIV (AIDS)   A person whose immune system has been infected by the human immunodeficiency virus (HIV) risks developing AIDS, Acquired Immune Deficiency Syndrome, for which no cure exists. The virus is transmitted by unprotected sexual contact with a carrier; by sharing contaminated needles; or during pregnancy, birth, or breastfeeding. About one out of four babies born to HIV-infected mothers will catch the virus, which can be detected by three to six months of age. Most affected children develop AIDS before turning six.

The risk of newborn infection can be minimized by giving the drug AZT to the mother during pregnancy and her baby at birth; by avoiding exposing the fetus and newborn to the mother's blood; and by feeding formula rather than breast milk. Careful treatment can also extend the mother's life by many years.

Your caregiver can advise you about testing for HIV before or during pregnancy. Or contact the National AIDS Hotline (see "Resources").

LISTERIOSIS   This bacterial infection, which causes flu-like symptoms in the mother, can trigger a baby's preterm birth, stillbirth, or meningitis (brain inflammation). To prevent listeriosis, avoid unpasteurized milk; soft cheeses such as brie, Camembert, Roquefort, feta, and Mexican-style soft cheeses; raw seafood; and undercooked meat.

LYME DISEASE   This infection, carried by deer ticks, can be transmitted to your baby during pregnancy. Doctors formerly believed that contracting Lyme disease in pregnancy could cause significant neurologic problems in the fetus, but recent studies suggest this isn't so. Lyme disease can make you very sick, however, so let your caregiver know if you think you've been bitten by a tick or if you notice a blotchy bull's-eye rash on your skin. If you are diagnosed with Lyme disease, you will probably receive antibiotics. You can limit your risk of catching this unpleasant disease by taking simple precautions:

▲ In wooded or grassy areas, wear long pants, long sleeves, and socks, and use a tick repellent.

▲ After hiking or camping, carefully check your skin for ticks, and take a shower.

▲ Inspect your dog for ticks after romps in the woods, and consult your vet about preventive measures.

RUBELLA (GERMAN MEASLES) A mild disease in children and adults, rubella can have tragic effects on a fetus whose mother catches the disease. If the mother is infected during the first trimester, possible fetal problems include deafness, heart disease, and cataracts.

Most pregnant women are immune to rubella, thanks to the vaccinations they received as children. Women who lack immunity can be vaccinated as adults, but should avoid conceiving for three months afterward. If you aren't immune, keep away from anyone who has rubella and let your caregiver know immediately if you've been exposed to this illness.

SEXUALLY TRANSMITTED DISEASES (STDS) These diseases include chlamydia (see page 108), condyloma (genital warts), gonorrhea, herpes (see page 110), human immunodeficiency virus (HIV, see page 111), and syphilis. STDs can seriously jeopardize your baby before, during, or soon after birth. Fortunately, routine screening, prompt treatment—usually with an antibiotic—and preventive measures, such as using a condom when you have sex, offer your baby protection during pregnancy. Genital warts, which often grow during pregnancy, should be medically treated to decrease bleeding and other complications at delivery. Because STDs may cause few if any symptoms, let your caregiver know if you have had many sexual partners or if you experience these symptoms:

▲ abnormal vaginal discharge;
▲ genital sores; or
▲ difficulty urinating.

TOXOPLASMOSIS   This protozoan infection sometimes causes flu-like symptoms in children and adults. When a woman catches it for the first time during pregnancy, it can result in miscarriage, prematurity, stillbirth, neonatal death, birth defects, and mental retardation. Sources of infection include undercooked meat, poultry, and fish, and cat feces. To avoid contracting toxoplasmosis, follow the precautions on pages 57 and 76.

WEST NILE VIRUS   Mosquitoes transmit this life-threatening infection. When a pregnant woman is infected, her fetus can become seriously ill. If you live in an area where there is West Nile Virus, use window screens and, when outdoors, wear protective clothing and mosquito repellent.

Infertility Problems

Most infertile couples who succeed in getting pregnant experience no related problems in pregnancy. But women with a history of infertility do run a slightly greater risk of miscarriage. Factors contributing to this increase include—

- ▲ a higher rate of multiple births due to fertility drugs,
- ▲ the hormonal or structural problems that caused the infertility, and
- ▲ the manipulation of eggs or embryos during technologically-assisted reproduction.

The good news is: Once a pregnancy is well established with a robust heartbeat and normal early fetal development, odds are great that this hard-won pregnancy will have a joyous outcome.

Multiple Birth

About one in 80 pregnancies results in the birth of more than one baby. Twins occur most frequently; triplets, quadruplets, and quintuplets are rare.

Identical twins, accounting for about one out of three twin births, result when a single egg fertilized by a single sperm divides into two embryos at an early stage. Because these twins have the same genetic inheritance, they look alike, share the same blood type, and are always the same sex. Identical twins occur at the same rate—about four sets per 1,000 births—all over the world.

Fraternal twins, accounting for two out of three twin pairs, result when two separate eggs are fertilized by two different sperm. These are the kind of twins that run in families. Just like any other pair of siblings, fraternal twins may or may not look alike. Half are same-sex twins, and half are opposite-sex twins. Certain characteristics make a mother more likely to bear fraternal twins or other multiples:

- ▲ being older (rates rise through a woman's thirties, drop slightly between 40 and 44, then rise sharply between 45 and 54);
- ▲ being black (blacks have the highest rate of fraternal twins, Asians have the lowest rate, and whites lie in between);
- ▲ having experienced several previous pregnancies;
- ▲ having previously given birth to twins;
- ▲ having used of birth control pills shortly before pregnancy;
- ▲ having used in-vitro fertilization or fertility drugs; and
- ▲ being a fraternal twin or having a close female relative who is the mother of fraternal twins.

You or your caregiver may suspect you are carrying more than one baby if a listener hears more than one heartbeat, if your uterus is bigger than expected or is growing very fast, or if you feel much more movement than with previous pregnancies. An ultrasound examination can confirm the diagnosis.

Having twins is exciting and scary. You'll need to gain more weight—35 to 45 pounds—and may feel pregnancy's discomforts sooner and more strongly than a woman expecting only one baby.

Prematurity poses the most serious medical risk to multiple pregnancy: Twins usually arrive about three weeks early, while triplets and quadruplets come even earlier. Because of this increased risk, you'll have more frequent examinations and will probably spend more of your pregnancy resting.

A woman expecting twins needs to make some extra preparation. Be sure you know the signs that labor has started (see pages 164 and 168). Prepare yourself for a possible cesarean; about half of twin deliveries are cesareans (see page 142). After the birth, you'll need all the help you can get. See "Resources" for information about helpful organizations to contact.

Phenylketonuria (PKU)

Since the 1960s, routine medical screening has identified newborns with a rare but potentially devastating condition. One in ten thousand babies cannot digest an amino acid called phenylalanine. In order to prevent the mental retardation that results when phenylalanine accumulates, parents of babies with PKU must provide them a phenylalanine-restricted diet.

Though women who were born with PKU may have long since abandoned dietary restrictions, high blood levels of phenylalanine during pregnancy could result in a baby with mental retardation or heart defects. That's why experts advise women with PKU to maintain a low-phenylalanine diet throughout their childbearing years. A pregnant woman with PKU should certainly avoid foods containing the artificial sweetener aspartame (Nutrasweet), which contains phenylalanine.

Preeclampsia and Eclampsia

Formerly called toxemia, preeclampsia is characterized by high blood pressure (see "Hypertension," page 106); swelling or puffiness of the hands and face along with sudden, rapid weight gain; and the presence of protein in the urine. Affecting about 6 percent of pregnancies, preeclampsia rarely occurs before the twentieth week. The cause remains a mystery. Any expectant mother can get preeclampsia. But these conditions raise a woman's risk:

- ▲ age under 20 or over 35
- ▲ being pregnant for the first time
- ▲ obesity
- ▲ poor nutrition
- ▲ having had preeclampsia in a previous pregnancy
- ▲ having a close female relative who experienced preeclampsia
- ▲ high blood pressure
- ▲ a kidney disorder
- ▲ autoimmune disorder, such as lupus, multiple sclerosis, or rheumatoid arthritis
- ▲ diabetes
- ▲ a seizure disorder

Regular checks of blood pressure, weight, and urine help catch this mysterious disease of pregnancy in its early stages, when it can be treated, usually with bed rest. Salt restriction is no longer considered a prevention or treatment for preeclampsia. If treatment fails to reverse preeclampsia, labor may be induced or a cesarean performed. The mother's blood pressure usually returns to normal shortly after the delivery.

Untreated preeclampsia can cause permanent damage to a mother's nervous system, blood vessels, or kidneys. Her baby can suffer growth retardation or oxygen deprivation. Preeclampsia sometimes progresses to **eclampsia,** in which a mother experiences convulsions, coma, and occasionally even death. Fortunately, eclampsia occurs in only one pregnancy in one thousand.

These symptoms could indicate that a mild case of preeclampsia may be progressing to a dangerous stage and should be reported to your caregiver:

▲ headaches
▲ blurred vision
▲ irritability
▲ breathlessness
▲ severe stomach pain, nausea, or vomiting

Rh and Other Blood Incompatibilities

If a baby's incompatible blood crosses the placenta during pregnancy or delivery, a mother may produce antibodies that attack her baby's red blood cells. Many newborns used to die as a result of blood incompatibilities, but today these problems can be prevented or treated.

The most serious blood incompatibility has to do with the Rh factor, named after a group of blood components first studied in rhesus monkeys. About nine out of ten people carry the Rh factor; they are called Rh-positive. Rh incompatibility poses a threat to a baby only if the mother is Rh-negative, *and* the baby's genetic father is Rh-positive, *and* the baby is Rh-positive (a baby may be Rh-negative even if his genetic father is Rh-positive).

An Rh-negative mother will receive injections of Rh immune globulin (RhoGam) at 28 weeks of pregnancy, to be repeated shortly after birth if her baby is Rh positive. RhoGam should also be given following any prenatal procedure during which the mother may be exposed to fetal blood, such as chorionic villus sampling (see page 38). The timely use of RhoGam prevents the mother from producing antibodies that attack her baby's blood.

Tests are also performed during pregnancy to determine whether a mother has become sensitized to the Rh factor, usually because of a previous medical transfusion or other exposure to Rh-positive blood. Sensitization can threaten a baby with jaundice, anemia, heart failure, and brain damage. Tests such as amniocentesis (see page 39) or percutaneous umbilical blood sampling (see page 39) can determine the extent of damage to fetal blood cells. An affected fetus or newborn may receive one or more blood transfusions (see "Percutaneous Umbilical Blood Sampling," page 39).

ABO incompatibility arises when a mother has type O blood and her partner has type A or B. Though this incompatibility occurs more commonly than Rh incompatibility, its effect—mild to moderate jaundice—is typically limited to the baby's first few days and is easily treated with exposure to bright lights and increased fluids. Only in rare cases is a transfusion needed.

Seizure Disorder (Epilepsy)

A condition that affects about 1 percent of pregnant women, epilepsy is linked to a higher rate of birth defects, including spina bifida and other neural tube problems. But the typical woman with a seizure disorder can look forward to a normal pregnancy and labor followed by delivery of a healthy baby.

Experts recommend delaying pregnancy until seizures are controlled by a minimal dosage of a single anticonvulsant medication. In addition, because seizure medications hamper folic acid metabolism, a woman with epilepsy will usually be advised to begin taking a daily dose of 4 milligrams of folic acid before conceiving. Higher levels of other vitamin supplements may be needed, too. Finally, because sleep deprivation increases the risk of having a seizure, a pregnant woman with seizure disorder should be sure to get plenty of rest.

Sickle Cell Disease

People with this inherited disorder have abnormal, sickle-shaped red blood cells that interfere with blood flow and can cause severe joint pain. Sickle cell disease can also lead to bone weakening, heart and kidney disease, and infections. One in about four hundred African Americans has sickle cell disease, which can be diagnosed at birth.

Pregnancy can worsen the symptoms, increasing the risk of miscarriage, stillbirth, and premature labor. If you have sickle cell disease you can have a healthy baby, but you must work closely with your medical caregivers. For example, you may require more frequent prenatal checkups. You may also receive transfusions during pregnancy, antibiotics at birth, or both. During pregnancy, you'll probably be told to avoid air travel, high-altitude vacations, and strenuous exercise.

If the baby's father carries the sickle cell trait, you will probably also be offered genetic counseling and screening, because your baby faces an increased risk for sickle cell disease.

Thyroid Disorders

For pregnancy to proceed normally, you need the right amount of thyroid hormone, which controls your body's metabolic rate and production of hormones. Women who have been diagnosed as having **hypothyroidism** (too little thyroid hormone) or **hyperthyroidism** (too much thyroid hormone) should be checked beforehand and frequently during pregnancy to make sure their medication dosages remain correct and that the medication they take is safe for pregnancy.

Well-controlled thyroid disorders have little effect on pregnancy. But untreated hyperthyroidism can seriously jeopardize the health of both mother and baby, raising the risk of miscarriage, low birth weight, preterm birth, and stillbirth. This disorder may strike suddenly during pregnancy. Symptoms of hyperthyroidism include excessive warmth, nervousness, a fast pulse and heart rate, extreme fatigue, diarrhea, and slow weight gain or even weight loss.

Untreated hypothyroidism can also put pregnancy in jeopardy, threatening miscarriage, fetal distress, and stillbirth. And recent research revealed that children whose mothers had untreated hypothyroidism later scored lower on IQ tests. Symptoms of hypothyroidism include fatigue, depression, intolerance of cold, muscle cramps, unexplained weight gain, and constipation.

Weight Problems

It's best to be at a healthy weight before beginning pregnancy. Being overweight increases a mother's risk of hypertension (see page 106), gestational diabetes (see page 104), preeclampsia (see page 115), and cesarean delivery. Her baby is also more likely to suffer neural tube defects or birth injuries.

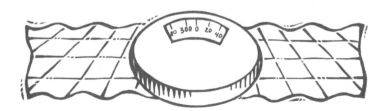

If you are obese at the start of pregnancy, don't go on a reducing diet, but do try to limit your weight gain to 10 to 15 pounds on a healthy, low-fat diet. Regular exercise may help you achieve this goal.

Women who are seriously underweight at the start of pregnancy run an increased risk of giving birth to a low-birth-weight or premature baby. If you are underweight, aim to attain your ideal body weight *plus* about 20 to 25 pounds (see page 45). Pile on the nourishing food, exercise moderately, and consider psychotherapy if you have an eating disorder.

Coping With a High-Risk Pregnancy

High-risk pregnancy could also be called high-stress pregnancy. All the stresses of a normal pregnancy get magnified when you have a risky medical condition to worry about.

Facing Your Feelings

Women going through a high-risk pregnancy commonly feel some or all of these feelings:

- ▲ anxiety about what might go wrong,
- ▲ resentment about the extra restrictions on their activity or increased dependency,
- ▲ guilt over actions they imagine may have caused the problem, and
- ▲ sadness about not having the pregnancy experience they anticipated.

Letting yourself express these normal feelings to your partner and close friends won't jinx your pregnancy or harm your baby. On the contrary, facing up honestly to these negative feelings may allow you to begin to feel hope.

Down But Not Out: Pregnancy on Bed Rest

Depending on your situation, you may have to restrict your activity or even stay in bed for some or most of your pregnancy. Be sure to get detailed instructions from your caregiver about what you should and shouldn't do. Women who have been confined to bed during pregnancy suggest the following:

- ▲ Choose the prettiest spot in the house.

When the Worst Happens: Pregnancy Loss

Whether in early pregnancy or after nine long months, losing a hoped-for baby is devastating. A baby's death kills her parents' dreams.

Surviving the Loss of Your Baby

There are many reasons that life sometimes ends before it begins. With increasing numbers of women undergoing prenatal screening and testing (see pages 34 to 40), more couples are making the difficult decision to end pregnancy because their babies have serious genetic defects. Planned termination can evoke as much grief as the natural loss of a wanted child, and the grief may be compounded by guilt over choosing to end the pregnancy. At least 20 percent of pregnancies end in miscarriage, and about 2 percent of pregnancies end early because they occur outside the uterus (see "Miscarriage and Ectopic Pregnancy," page 21). One in approximately two hundred babies dies after the twentieth week of pregnancy, when the baby is termed stillborn. Stillbirth may have no explanation, or may stem from genetic defects, maternal disease or infection, an umbilical cord accident, or placental abnormalities.

Parents generally know in advance that a baby will be stillborn. Usually, a doctor determines that the fetus has died and then induces labor, using prostaglandins (see page 167) and Pitocin (see page 138).

After the delivery, parents who suffer a stillbirth should be able to—

▲ see and hold the baby;
▲ name the baby;
▲ keep a photograph and a lock of hair;
▲ hold a memorial or funeral service;
▲ get their questions answered, if possible, about why the baby died;
▲ find support from professionals at the hospital or a high-risk maternity center; and
▲ seek solace from other parents who have lost a baby (see "Resources").

Even if they never get to hold their child, parents mourn the loss of a hoped-for baby. Feelings of distress and depression can linger for many months, long after acquaintances may expect the parents to feel better. Bereaved parents show their grief in different ways. One partner may want to cry and talk a lot, while the other may withdraw or act angry. Holding back these normal feelings can make it impossible to embrace each other, let alone the challenge of a new pregnancy.

Another Baby? Maybe

It takes courage to attempt pregnancy again after such a blow. If you decide to undertake another pregnancy, surround yourself with people who recognize and applaud your strength.

You may feel anxious before each milestone of the pregnancy. If you previously suffered an early miscarriage, you may worry only until you pass the point in pregnancy at which you miscarried. But if you experienced a stillbirth, no point in pregnancy may seem safe to you. Parents who have lost more than one baby may also feel frightened throughout a following pregnancy.

Your worries will probably alternate with more positive feelings. Indeed, many parents describe feeling scared and excited in turn or experiencing rushes of conflicting emotions.

It's only natural to restrain your excitement about having another baby after you've lost one. The normal urge to control a risky situation makes you want to do things differently during a subsequent pregnancy. You may—

▲ choose to learn as little or as much as possible about your new baby before the birth;

▲ focus a lot of energy on eating right and staying healthy;

▲ change the type of obstetric care you seek (for example, you may opt for more or less risk-oriented care);

▲ seek support at a local hospital, through an organization that matches you to a trained telephone volunteer, or via the Internet (see "Resources," pages 209 to 210);

▲ request more attention from your prenatal caregiver; and

▲ make extra prenatal visits just to be able to hear your baby's reassuring heartbeat.

Parents often wonder whether they will ever be able to love a new baby the way they loved the baby who died. In fact, most couples cope well with such a loss and move on to enjoy a subsequent child. But losing a wished-for baby forever changes you and the way you parent. Afterward, you may become a sadder, but wiser and more appreciative, parent. You'll learn that loving a new baby doesn't diminish your feelings for the one you lost. When you hold your new baby in your arms, you may feel some new fears and a wave of sadness, but you should also feel joy. If sad feelings continue to trouble you weeks after bringing your new baby home, you may want to seek professional counseling.

▲ Stow everything you need within arm's reach, including a telephone, a cooler for snacks, and a pitcher of ice water.

▲ Put up a calendar on which to mark your progress toward birth.

▲ Establish a daily schedule.

▲ Ask your partner or a friend to organize people to do chores, such as shopping, housecleaning, and laundry.

▲ Find out what exercises are permitted, perhaps seeing a physical therapist for guidance, and setting up a regular schedule of isometrics or other allowable toning exercises.

▲ Keep a diary, which might be the start of your baby's first scrapbook.

▲ Work on projects such as rearranging your photo albums, sorting through correspondence and other papers, writing letters, or cleaning up your recipe file.

▲ Become expert in some area, such as old movies or a favorite kind of music.

▲ Knit or crochet something special for your baby.

▲ Do something you have long put off, such as learning a foreign language.

▲ Link up with another mother who is also experiencing a high-risk pregnancy (see "Resources").

▲ Arrange private childbirth classes.

Working with Your Prenatal Caregiver

If you're confined to bed rest, your prenatal visits may become your only outings. Your caregiver can be a valuable source of information as well as support. Be sure to:

▲ Let your caregiver know exactly what you need.

▲ Write down questions as they occur to you and bring them to your appointments.

▲ Ask for medical explanations in simple language.

▲ Take notes.

▲ Ask for written sources if you need more information on any subject.

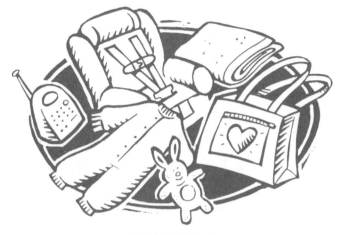

CHAPTER 7

Preparing to Have Your Baby

As you get closer to your due date, your thoughts will naturally turn toward labor, delivery, and bringing your baby home. The next sections offer information about these and other issues. Be sure to note any questions you'd like to discuss with your caregiver.

Childbirth Classes

In general, women who take childbirth classes use less medication, have fewer forceps deliveries, and feel better about their babies' births than women who don't take classes. No matter how you feel about medication and other birth interventions, a good childbirth class should help you sort out your choices and feel more knowledgeable about the big event to come. Even if you took a childbirth class during a prior pregnancy, you may benefit from a refresher course. And if you're homebound, a teacher may be willing to come to you.

> **Your Due Date Approaches** You'll probably find yourself thinking more about questions like these:
>
> *What kind of childbirth class should I take?*
>
> *Should I take classes on infant care?*
>
> *How will I feed my baby?*
>
> *Should I have electronic fetal monitoring or other obstetric procedures during labor?*
>
> *Can I avoid an episiotomy?*
>
> *Should I have natural childbirth or choose medication such as an epidural?*
>
> *What people would I like to accompany me to the birth?*
>
> *What will birth be like if I need a cesarean?*
>
> *Should I have my baby boy circumcised?*
>
> *Who will be my baby's doctor?*
>
> *Will I need help at home after the baby comes?*

What You Need to Know

A good childbirth class offers two important things: emotional support and information. The support comes from the teacher and from other expectant parents, with whom you'll be able to share your discomforts, fears, and hopes. The information should cover, at the very least, the normal progress of labor, vaginal and cesarean birth, hospital (or birth center, or homebirth) procedures, relaxation, pain management, and newborn care. Many classes also include topics such as prenatal exercises, nutrition, and breastfeeding. In addition to or instead of a standard childbirth class, you may choose to take a class more specifically targeted for people expecting twins, a cesarean, or a vaginal birth after cesarean (see "VBAC," page 146). Standard classes are intended for couples, so plan to attend with your partner or the person who will accompany you in labor. If you plan to have a doula at the birth (see page 151) in addition to your partner, the doula should also be welcome in class.

WHEN SHOULD YOU TAKE CHILDBIRTH CLASSES? Depending on where you live, you may be able to sign up for an early-bird class which will concentrate on nutrition and exercise. Bradley teachers (see page 126) offer one early class, followed by weekly classes from the sixth month on. Lamaze classes (see below) usually begin in the seventh month and end about three weeks before a mother's due date. Depending on what topics your childbirth classes include, you may want to take an extra class on breast-feeding or baby care in your last trimester.

WHAT DO CLASSES COST? Fees for classes vary widely by location, from free to a price tag of $250 or more. The bigger your city, the more your childbirth classes will probably cost. A few insurance companies and health-maintenance organizations offer partial or full reimbursement for the class fees, because they consider childbirth classes good preventive medicine. Be sure to ask.

In general, private instructors charge more than hospitals, many of which offer inexpensive or free childbirth classes. But hospital-sponsored programs aren't always a bargain. Although they can familiarize you with the hospital setting, each class may have 12 or more couples in attendance. That's probably too many to allow enough time for assisted practice in childbirth techniques such as relaxation. In addition, an instructor employed by the hospital may hesitate to give objective information about birth interventions (see pages 135 to 151). In contrast, independent childbirth teachers, even if they hold classes in a hospital, usually plan their own curriculum and determine class size. Whether you choose a hospital-sponsored or independent program, make sure that your classes are small enough to allow individual attention and that the instructor plans to cover the topics you would like to learn.

WHAT ARE THE MAIN METHODS? Childbirth organizations teach various techniques of managing pain and avoiding complications in labor. Certification by a local or national professional childbirth organization means that a teacher has met minimum standards, including supervised teaching. The largest such certifying organizations are Lamaze International; the American Academy of Husband-Coached Childbirth, for the Bradley Method; and the International Childbirth Education Association (see "Resources").

Lamaze classes emphasize concentration based on relaxation, promoted by breathing patterns that are much simpler and slower than the parodies you've probably seen at the movies and on TV. During labor, Lamaze-prepared women direct their attention to a focal point, which may be something to look at, listen to, feel, or imagine. Classes include instruction on positions and body movements that promote comfort during labor. Lamaze partners learn verbal coaching and massage techniques to reduce pain even further. Teachers explain the pros and cons of medication and other interventions and encourage students to talk with their caregivers in order to make well-informed decisions. Classes, taught in a series of two to six sessions, typically total about 12 hours. Intensive weekend Lamaze classes have become popular in some areas.

Emphasizing relaxation through an inward focus, **Bradley** classes cover many types of relaxation, so the laboring woman can use what works best for her. Unlike their Lamaze counterparts, Bradley instructors don't teach specific breathing patterns, but instead encourage a woman to relax and breathe normally. The American Academy of Husband-Coached Childbirth, which trains Bradley teachers, strongly discourages the use of medication and other interventions during labor. Though labor coaches are usually husbands, Bradley teachers help women without husbands or partners to find alternative coaches. Bradley classes typically consist of 12 two-hour sessions. Many are taught at home by married couples, and class size is generally small.

ICEA teachers don't all teach a particular method, but instead stress "freedom of choice based on a knowledge of alternatives." ICEA-certified teachers may teach patterned breathing as well as other relaxation techniques. Like Lamaze teachers, ICEA teachers encourage their students to make informed decisions about medication and interventions.

Finding the Class for You

Childbirth educators differ not only in which organizations certify them and whether or not they are hospital employees. They also have had different experiences as parents, teachers, and labor companions. Many teachers incorporate ideas gleaned outside their formal training. So plan to do some research to find the right teacher for you.

To locate a childbirth educator you like, ask your birth attendant, look in the Yellow Pages, or talk to friends who have babies.

> **Childbirth Classes** In addition to finding out about dates and times, class size, location, and fees, you may want to ask the teacher some of these questions:

How long have you been teaching childbirth classes?

What pain-relieving methods do you teach?

How much time will the class spend practicing various pain-relieving techniques?

What do you think about the use of drugs in labor?

Will you give advice on reducing the risk for cesarean section and other interventions?

Do you offer private classes for housebound parents or a refresher course for experienced parents?

Do you cover breastfeeding and other postpartum concerns?

Could your family benefit from prenatal classes, too? Some communities offer special classes to prepare grandparents and siblings (see page 152) for the arrival of the newest family member.

— ♥ —

Classes on Infant Care

A generation ago, parents learned about their newborns in the course of leisurely hospital stays that averaged four or five days for a vaginal birth and a week for cesarean. No longer. In 1995, hospital stays averaged less than two days for vaginal birth and about four days for cesarean. For this reason, you and your partner may want to take classes on infant care before your baby is born.

Even if you're experienced with babies, some baby-care basics have changed recently. For example, since 1992 the American Academy of Pediatrics has recommended placing infants to sleep on their backs. This simple change has cut deaths from Sudden Infant Death Syndrome (SIDS) by 38 percent.

Many hospitals and birthing centers provide such classes on general baby care, on breastfeeding, and on infant CPR (cardiopulmonary resuscitation). You can also find baby-care classes through your caregiver or childbirth teacher, your YMCA, the American Red Cross local parenting organizations, or the Yellow Pages.

———❤———
Taking a Strong Position

Because no one position is best for labor and birth, practice your pain-relieving techniques in several different ones. Some obstetrical practices—for example, intravenous medications, electronic fetal monitoring, and epidural anesthesia—can interfere with a woman's freedom to move. So be sure to talk to your caregiver in advance if you want to try different positions during labor. Ask which ones are possible, which are encouraged, and whether your birthing place offers positional aids such as a birthing ball or squatting bar.

As you labor, you'll soon discover which positions are most comfortable, which help you relax, and which speed your labor along. Avoid prolonged lying on your back. In addition to impairing circulation and causing back pain, back-lying can slow labor because the uterus naturally tilts forward when it contracts. Usually, the most comfortable positions are those that allow the uterus to tip away from the spine.

If your labor lasts for many hours, you'll probably want to alternate between positions that help you relax and those that promote the progress of labor. The all-fours position, for example, offers the added benefit of encouraging your baby to get into position for birth, facing your back. Squatting can widen your pelvis for an easier delivery.

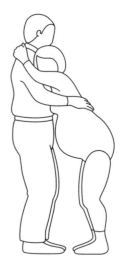

▲ Standing, leaning, and walking let you work with gravity, making contractions more effective and less painful, easing back pain, and perhaps speeding labor. Your partner can support you as if you were partners in a dance marathon.

▲ Sitting up straight or leaning back is relaxing and uses gravity to encourage the baby to descend. But leaning back can also increase back pain. If that happens, try straddling a chair, leaning forward on a pillow.

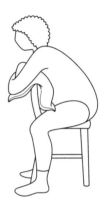

▲ Side-lying is relaxing, enhances circulation to the uterus, reduces blood pressure, and eases back pain.

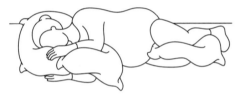

▲ Squatting uses gravity, eases back pain, widens the pelvic opening, and presses the baby's head down. Between contractions, rest in a sitting or kneeling position.

▲ Kneeling as you lean forward uses gravity and eases back pain. Kneeling with your thighs resting on your calves widens the pelvic opening and presses the baby's head down.

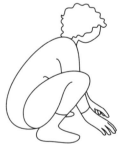
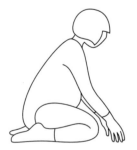

▲ Kneeling with one leg and squatting with the other uses gravity and eases back pain.

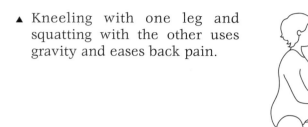

▲ Getting on all fours eases back pain and may encourage the baby's head to rotate into position for birth. This position can also help the birth of a baby with large shoulders and reduce your risk of perineal tearing. Don't sag, though. Instead, keep your back flat or arched up slightly.

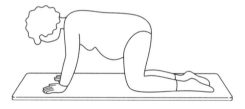

──♥── Touring the Hospital

Even if you've already explored your hospital or birthing center, you may want to take another tour closer to your delivery date. This tour should offer you a good idea of the kind of help you can expect from the labor and delivery nurses, who provide the main source of medical support during a hospital labor.

If your caregiver doesn't have hospital preregistration forms, ask the leader of your hospital tour about them. Filling out insurance forms in advance ensures that your partner can stay with you and not be preoccupied with paperwork when you need support during labor.

Be sure, too, to find out where to park when you arrive in labor, and how to get to the labor-and-delivery ward quickly.

Hospital or Birthing Center Tour You should find out what supplies the facility provides and what you'll need to bring from home. You might ask:

Do you have a tape or CD player that I can use to play relaxing music during labor?

Should I bring extra pillows for comfort during labor?

Will you offer juice, tea, and Popsicles, or should I bring my own?

Do you have beepers for loan or rent so I can get in touch with my birth partner when I go into labor?

See page 9 for other questions to ask about policies for labor and postpartum care.

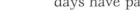

The Feeding Choice

Breast, bottle, or a combination of the two? This is a big decision. To make an informed choice, you'll need to get the facts and explore your feelings. Making a choice you feel good about will help you enjoy feeding times, which are a huge part of caring for a newborn. Be sure to enlist your partner's support for your decisions; recent research revealed that three out of four infants whose fathers supported nursing were breastfed, compared with fewer than one out of ten infants whose fathers held no opinion. Not sure which choice to make? Try nursing. It's much easier to switch to bottle feeding than it is to initiate nursing after a few days have passed.

Breast Is Best

Currently, about seven out of ten women in the United States choose to breastfeed. You probably know that your milk is the best food for your baby and the only food she needs for the first four to six months. Breastfed babies suffer fewer ear infections, colds, food allergies, and hospitalizations than do formula-fed babies.

Nursing promotes better jaw and tooth development. It also reduces the risk of future health problems, such as asthma, childhood leukemia, type I diabetes, lymphoma, and Crohn's disease. Recent studies have even related breastfeeding to reduced obesity and better intellectual development in children.

As a nursing mother, you'll get your own rewards. Oxytocin, a hormone released when the milk lets down, contracts your uterus and minimizes postpartum bleeding. Another breastfeeding hormone, prolactin, promotes motherly behavior and relaxes you. Studies suggest that breastfeeding can reduce a woman's future risk for breast cancer and osteoporosis. Compared with the cost of formula feeding, nursing will save you hundreds of dollars a year. It's convenient, too: no formula to buy, no bottles to sterilize and heat, and nothing to mix or measure in the middle of the night. Best of all, perhaps, nursing lets you consume 400 to 500 extra calories a day and still lose weight!

The emotional benefits of nursing can't be measured, but breastfeeding will bring you and your newborn as close as you can be. Because you have to hold your baby to nurse, breastfeeding makes for a strong attachment between the two of you. That mother-child bond will give your baby an irreplaceable sense of love, security, and warmth.

Getting Ready to Nurse

Having a premature baby, a cesarean, or twins needn't keep you from breastfeeding. Neither should returning to work right away. With determination and support, you can nurse successfully even in these challenging situations.

You needn't make complicated preparations to nurse, such as rubbing your nipples. Here are a few simple things to do instead:

▲ Let your caregiver and the baby's doctor know you plan to nurse.

▲ Read a good book on breastfeeding (see "Further Reading").

▲ Take a breastfeeding class.

▲ Find supporters: friends and family members who have nursed, for example, and a local La Leche League leader, or a local lactation consultant (see "Resources").

▲ Avoid using soap on your nipples; it dries and irritates them.

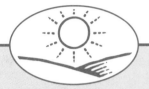

Don't Want to Nurse? Reasons to Reconsider

"I had problems nursing my first baby."
You may not have problems with this baby.

"I don't think I'll like it."
Try it. You'll probably be surprised by how pleasant and easy it is, and you can always stop if it doesn't work out.

"I'm too small- or large-busted to nurse."
Milk production is independent of breast size.

"I've had breast surgery."
Check with your surgeon, but modern breast surgery techniques often allow women to nurse.

"I have to go back to work."
Even a few weeks of nursing offers you and baby a great start. When you go back to work, you can pump milk and leave it for your baby, and/or you can nurse her at night.

"My family isn't supportive."
A family member who doesn't support breastfeeding may not understand what's best for you and your baby. Stand up for yourself and your baby, and do what's best for both of you.

"My partner wants to help feed the baby."
Your partner can help by feeding the baby a bottle of pumped breast milk or formula once in a while or by getting the baby ready for you to nurse.

▲ Make sure your nipples stick out so that your baby can latch on and suck them (see page 24).

The Downside of Nursing

At first, breastfeeding may seem like more trouble than bottle feeding. The perfect digestibility of breast milk means you need to feed your baby more often than you would with formula, especially at the very beginning. Many nursing mothers experience a few days of nipple soreness. More serious problems, such as extremely sore or cracked nipples, clogged milk ducts, and breast infections, occur sometimes. Each of these problems can be prevented or treated.

Because nursing is a dance for two, other family members may feel left out. Invite them to join in by offering the baby an occasional bottle of pumped breast milk or formula. To get your baby used to a bottle, it's best to introduce it at about three to four weeks. Give yourself this time to establish your milk supply and build up your confidence at breastfeeding. If you wait much longer than a month, you may find that your baby balks at any substitutes.

While nursing, you'll need to eat well and avoid strict reducing diets, smoking, excessive alcohol drinking, and drugs that might harm the baby. Working mothers must make special arrangements to pump and store milk at work, or combine nursing with formula feeding.

Few illnesses and medications need spell an end to nursing. But you should avoid breastfeeding if you have HIV or if you need to undergo chemical or radiation treatment for cancer.

Bottle Feeding with Love

Of course, babies can thrive on formula, too. Mothers who plan to return to work very quickly or who intend to go on a strict reducing diet sometimes choose bottle feeding. Some mothers, or their partners, simply feel more comfortable feeding their babies by bottle. Once you make your choice, let go of guilt, and concentrate on the other important aspects of mothering. Before your baby is born, ask the doctor or family practitioner what type of formula, bottles, and nipples to buy and how many of each you'll need. Since your baby may show a preference for a particular formula or nipple shape, it's best not to purchase too many of these items beforehand.

Birth Options

The role technology, medication, staff members, and labor companions will play at your baby's hospital birth depends partly on medical need and partly on the way things are usually done. But your own preferences and the agreements you work out beforehand with your prenatal caregiver will also affect the use of interventions at your birth.

As you read this section on birth options, note questions and concerns so that you can discuss them with your partner and birth attendant before labor begins. Although you can't script your baby's birth, you should certainly say how you'd like things to go.

Birth Technology

The technology used during labor and birth may comfort you, or it may make you more anxious. Keep in mind that most of the interventions described below are useful in certain situations.

Obstetrics is an unpredictable field, and true emergencies, although rare, do occur. In a case of severe fetal distress or major maternal bleeding, for example, you could end up with an emergency forceps delivery or a cesarean section performed by your own caregiver or a doctor you've never met if your caregiver is unavailable. In an emergency there is little time to answer questions, and the mother has few choices. But even if an emergency dictates a change in your plans for birth, you and your partner should have plenty of time afterward to discuss with your caregiver exactly what happened, what was done, and why. A thorough explanation should help you both adjust to an unexpected turn of events.

In fact, most obstetrical interventions—the use of forceps, episiotomies, the administration of Pitocin, and cesarean deliveries—are used in nonemergency situations. You and your birth partner have the right to be fully informed about the risks and benefits of any nonemergency interventions and to let your caregiver know whether you want various procedures preferred.

PREP AND ENEMA   The prep—shaving a woman's pubic and perineal hair—used to be performed for two reasons. Doctors thought that bacteria clung to pubic hair and that shaving would keep hair out of the episiotomy site (see "Episiotomy," page 139). But the shave hurt, and the pubic hair itched as it grew back. Too, research showed that shaving actually increased the infection rate, because of tiny razor nicks.

If you need an episiotomy, you may receive a minimal clip or shave of the hairs right on your perineum. Most caregivers skip this.

For years, women found enemas an uncomfortable part of giving birth. Now at most hospitals the enema is optional, not routine. Advocates of the procedure claimed three benefits—that an enema stimulated uterine contractions, made room for the baby's head, and reduced contamination of the delivery area. But taking an enema doesn't always shorten labor or keep the delivery area clean. In one study, enemas made no difference in the length of labor or in whether or not women passed stool during birth.

Because most women have frequent loose bowel movements just before labor or early in the process, an enema is usually unnecessary. But some women feel uncomfortable pushing if they think they may move their bowels. If you haven't had a bowel movement for at least a day when labor begins, you might ask your caregiver whether you should give yourself an enema or use a painless glycerin suppository at home; you can buy either at a drugstore. Or ask the hospital nurse for an enema, if you think that it will make you feel more comfortable.

ELECTRONIC FETAL MONITORING   The fetal monitor, a machine that resembles a videocassette recorder, simultaneously registers your contractions and your baby's heartbeat, to indicate how your baby is responding to labor. High-risk, medicated, or Pitocin-enhanced labors should be monitored electronically.

Fetal monitoring can be done externally or internally. **External monitoring** uses two belts around the mother's abdomen. The top belt has a pressure-sensitive gauge that reacts to the changing shape of the belly as the uterus contracts, then relaxes. Since contractions begin at the top of the uterus but are felt only when they reach the cervix a few seconds later, some women like to use the monitor printout to cue their relaxation and breathing at the beginning of each contraction. The second belt, worn near the groin, contains an ultrasound device that registers the opening and closing of the baby's heart valves. If you change positions or your baby moves a lot, this belt may need frequent repositioning.

Occasionally **internal monitoring** is used to get a more accurate recording. For this procedure, the amniotic sac must be ruptured (see "Amniotomy," page 139) and the cervix at least 2 centimeters dilated. A tiny spiral electrode is nudged 1 to 2 millimeters under the baby's scalp, providing an EKG, or electrocardiogram, reading of the baby's heartbeat. Contractions are also monitored, either internally by the insertion of a tiny catheter into the uterus, or externally with the abdominal belt. In a twin birth, after the bag of water breaks, the bottom twin is usually monitored internally and the top twin externally.

Many parents find electronic monitoring reassuring, and some caregivers prefer to use it for all births, not just high-risk cases. But even though you can change positions during monitoring, and should be encouraged to do so, the attachments may make you feel as if you should remain on your side.

Medical research has uncovered two other problems with routine fetal monitoring. First, for low-risk mothers, electronic monitoring has shown no benefit over the old-fashioned method of listening to the baby's heart tones with a fetoscope. Second, after its rise in the late 1970s, continuous monitoring contributed to a surge in cesarean deliveries, probably because monitored mothers were instructed to lie on their backs during labor and because the readings were hard to interpret and often caused undue alarm.

Responding to this research, the American College of Obstetricians and Gynecologists concluded in 1988 that intermittent listening **(ausculation)** with a stethoscope or Doppler ultrasound device is an acceptable alternative for low-risk mothers. But you may not be offered this option unless your hospital has one-to-one nursing care or you're being attended by a nurse-midwife or a private-duty nurse who is willing to ausculate you throughout your entire labor. In fact, in 2002, over 85 percent of mothers were monitored electronically during labor.

If you'd prefer to stay active during labor, ask whether you can have electronic monitoring only during your first half hour in the hospital and then intermittently—about 15 minutes out of each hour. Ask, too, whether your hospital offers radio **telemetry,** which would allow you to stroll around the vicinity of your labor room while your baby's heart rate is monitored. Similar to a cordless phone, the telemetry monitor can be clipped to your gown.

INTRAVENOUS SOLUTION (IV)   You'll probably receive IV fluids—which are usually sugar and water—if you experience excessive vomiting, dehydration, or exhaustion; if your baby appears stressed (fluids boost placental circulation); or if you face an increased risk of bleeding. Pitocin (see page 138) is usually given via an intravenous infusion. An IV is also routine when a mother asks for a shot of narcotics or an epidural (see "Medication," page 149). Medications, especially the epidural, tend to lower maternal blood pressure, and IV fluids can help keep it at a healthy level.

Some birth attendants believe all women in labor should be on an IV in order to keep a vein open in case of an emergency. But a heparin lock—a tiny needle containing heparin, an anti-coagulant—can also keep your vein open. If necessary, a plug on the end of the needle can later be inserted into an IV line. A heparin lock lets you walk around more easily than if you needed to wheel around an IV apparatus.

You may be given an IV simply to supply fluids during labor. But you shouldn't need an IV if your labor is normal and you can keep down clear fluids, such as water, tea, or juice.

PITOCIN   When your baby is ready to be born, signals received from your baby and your body cause your pituitary gland to release oxytocin, a hormone that stimulates uterine contractions. At times, this natural process requires a medical nudge to begin or continue. For example, your baby may be overdue, or waiting for labor may be considered unsafe because of your condition or the baby's. Pitocin, synthetic oxytocin, is commonly used when membranes rupture and labor fails to begin on its own. It may also be used when labor is prolonged. If you need Pitocin, synthetic oxytocin, you'll get it through an IV in carefully controlled doses. Your labor must then be monitored electronically because Pitocin can cause very strong contractions. For this reason the U.S. Food and Drug Administration requires that Pitocin be used only when medically necessary for the safety of mother or baby.

Pitocin can shorten labor. But it also produces strong contractions that can peak suddenly. To cope with a Pitocin-induced labor, try these tips:

▲ Ask your partner to watch the fetal monitor or keep a hand on the top of your abdomen to let you know when a contraction is beginning. This way you can be ready with your breathing and relaxation techniques.

▲ Adapt the breathing and relaxation patterns you learned in childbirth class to cope with the sudden onset of pain. For example, instead of taking a long cleansing breath at the beginning of a contraction, think "release," and breathe out first.

▲ If you feel able to walk around between contractions, doing so may help you cope with the pain. Ask to be monitored by telemetry (see page 137).

▲ Remember that Pitocin can make labor shorter and harder. Labor may progress faster than you thought possible.

Because Pitocin works best when the cervix is effaced and somewhat dilated, your caregiver may first use prostaglandin, in the form of a gel or tablet (see page 167), to ready your cervix for induction. The use of prostaglandin reduces induction failures, lowering the rate of cesareans for "failure to progress." But because prostaglandin as well as Pitocin can trigger strong contractions, and because prostaglandin gel may increase the risk of uterine rupture in a vaginal birth following a cesarean (see page 146), you should be given these agents only under careful observation. Be sure to discuss the risks and benefits of these medications with your caregivers before they are used.

Pitocin is also frequently used after birth to minimize postpartum bleeding by strengthening uterine contractions.

AMNIOTOMY   Your bag of waters can break naturally at any time before or during labor. It may remain intact until you begin pushing or even until your baby is born, or your caregiver may break it during labor in a procedure called amniotomy. Birth attendants perform this procedure with an instrument that looks like a long plastic crochet hook. Reports differ on whether amniotomy actually speeds labor. Other possible reasons for amniotomy are to examine the amniotic fluid, to insert an internal fetal monitor electrode (see "Electronic Fetal Monitoring," page 136), or to speed the birth of a second twin.

Critics of artificial membrane rupture argue that the fluid in the amniotic sac cushions the baby's head, preventing excessive molding of the baby's skull bones and pressure on the umbilical cord. Amniotomy with a baby in the breech position or when the head is high risks umbilical cord prolapse, is a grave emergency that makes a cesarean delivery necessary.

Though the procedure itself is painless, amniotomy can cause contractions to strengthen. To avoid infection, delivery should ideally take place within a few hours, so you may be given Pitocin after your membranes are ruptured.

The alternative to amniotomy? Unless there is a clear-cut benefit, let nature take its course.

EPISIOTOMY   This cut—usually down toward the anus, but occasionally on the diagonal—enlarges the vaginal opening just before birth and requires stitching under a local anesthetic afterward. Though 34 percent of women who gave birth in 2000 had episiotomies—a steep decline from 1980, when 64 percent were cut—caregivers' individual rates vary widely. Some caregivers perform episiotomies in less than 10 percent of the births they attend. Others cut and stitch more than 90 percent of first-time mothers in their care. With stretchier tissues, second-timers are more likely to avoid episiotomy.

Episiotomy has some medical advantages. The cut can speed delivery by a few minutes, a margin that may help a distressed baby or a tired mother. Episiotomy can help a big baby through a tight, muscular perineum; reduce pressure on the head of a fragile premie; or release a trapped head or shoulders. The cut can also ease the application of forceps and prevent painful tearing at the front of the vagina.

But research has shown that an episiotomy performed simply as a routine procedure—

- ▲ does *not* necessarily heal faster than a natural tear,
- ▲ may *not* decrease future pelvic floor muscle damage,
- ▲ does *not* reduce the risk of head injury when the baby is born at full term, and
- ▲ does *not* decrease the mother's risk of a severe tear that extends to the anus.

In fact, instead of preventing severe tears into the anus, routine episiotomies actually make them more likely. Why? Imagine ripping a sheet into rags. Tearing an uncut sheet is hard work. But snipping the edge first makes tearing the sheet easier.

When advised to restrain their pushing efforts, most women can deliver their babies over an intact perineum or with only minor tears. These naturally occurring tears may or may not need stitching. Stitched tears, especially when they're only skin deep, often heal more comfortably than an episiotomy, which cuts through muscle as well as skin.

Ask whether your caregiver uses any special methods to avoid episiotomy. In addition to patience, some midwives and doctors recommend delivery in gravity-employing positions, such as squatting, kneeling, or semi-squatting with support. These caregivers may provide warm compresses and soothing oils, and many also encourage practicing prenatal **perineal massage** about five minutes a day beginning about six weeks before the due date.

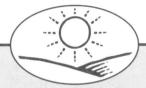

Perineal Massage

▲ Sit, leaning back, in bed. Or stand, with one foot resting on the seat of a chair.

▲ Lubricate your fingers with vegetable oil or a water-soluble gel, such as K-Y jelly.

▲ With your thumbs on the inside and other fingers on the outside, make a U-shaped movement around the portion of your vagina toward the back of your body.

▲ Apply just enough pressure to create a stinging sensation, while you focus on relaxing.

If you'd like to do this exercise with your partner, use the sitting position. Have him put his index fingers inside your vagina and his thumbs outside, and let him know how much pressure to apply.

If you have herpes or a vaginal infection, ask your caregiver whether you should do this exercise.

FORCEPS   These metal instruments for aiding a vaginal delivery look something like giant salad tongs. Forceps have two parts, which lock at their intersection so that the "blades" cannot squeeze the baby's head. These blades aren't sharp and they are curved to conform to the shape of the vagina and the baby's head.

Forceps may be used in the pushing stage of labor to speed the birth, if the baby's head is too big or in the wrong position to be born without help, or if the mother is unable to continue pushing. The delivery is called **high forceps** if the baby's head is unengaged in the pelvis, **mid-forceps** if the head is engaged but not visible, **low forceps** if the head is close to the vaginal opening, and **outlet forceps** if the head is stretching the perineum.

The higher in the birth canal that forceps are used, the more skill is required, and the greater is the risk of injury to baby and mother. High-forceps deliveries, which damaged tiny heads, shoulders, and arms, have disappeared in modern obstetrics. They have been replaced by safer cesarean deliveries.

When a baby is delivered by forceps the mother may need a larger episiotomy (see "Episiotomy," page 139) or extra stitches. Whether or not an episiotomy is performed, her risk for cervical and perineal tears increases. The baby may show facial bruises for a few days, or may not have any marks at all. Between 1990 and 2000, forceps use declined from 8.6 percent to 4 percent as the vacuum extractor gained popularity.

VACUUM EXTRACTOR   Like forceps, the vacuum extractor can give a mother assistance to push out her baby. Vacuum use climbed from 6.1 percent in 1990 to 8.4 percent in 2000. This device consists of a cap applied to the top of the baby's head and held in place by suction. When the caregiver pulls on a handle extending from the cap, the baby's head moves down.

In expert hands, the vacuum extractor is no more dangerous for the baby than forceps, though the suction may cause a temporary swelling and bruising on the top of the baby's head. Compared to using forceps, though, vacuum extraction means fewer tears, less pain, and less blood loss for mothers who need help with their deliveries. Because either vacuum or forceps use can cause rare but serious risks to babies, be sure to discuss management choices for a slow labor with your caregiver before the time comes.

Cesarean Birth

Currently just over one in four American births is a cesarean section. The delivery of a baby through a surgical cut in the abdomen and uterus, a cesarean can be a life-saving operation. But this major surgery also multiplies a mother's risks of infection, injury, and even death. It also lengthens the postpartum recovery and makes later deliveries a little riskier. For these reasons, a cesarean should be done only when the health of a mother or baby is in jeopardy.

WHEN IS A CESAREAN NECESSARY?   A mother may need a cesarean for—

- ▲ a labor that fails to progress because the cervix doesn't dilate completely or the baby doesn't descend;
- ▲ breech presentation;

▲ other abnormal presentation of the baby, such as side-lying;

▲ an irregular fetal heartbeat suggesting fetal distress that doesn't respond to a change in the mother's position or the administration of oxygen to the mother (Fetal scalp blood testing—or an experimental, noninvasive test called pulse oximetry, which uses a light sensor to check the baby's blood—can detect possible oxygen deprivation and confirm the need for a speedy delivery.);

▲ severe preeclampsia;

▲ twins or other multiples, when one or more of the babies is not in a head-down position;

▲ cord prolapse, when the cord falls into the vagina ahead of the baby's head or buttocks;

▲ placenta previa, in which the placenta blocks the cervical opening; or

▲ placental abruption, in which the placenta begins to separate from the uterus before the birth.

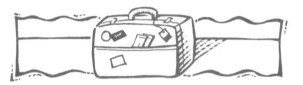

PREVENTING AN UNNECESSARY CESAREAN   Although a cesarean section can sometimes be the safest medical option for mother and baby, you can reduce your own chance of needing a cesarean. Here are some ways:

▲ If you can, stay active and avoid excessive weight gain during pregnancy. Physically active women of normal weight have lower cesarean rates than their sedentary, overweight sisters.

▲ Choose a caregiver who has a cesarean rate of under 20 percent and who recommends vaginal birth after cesarean (see "VBAC," page 146) for most women who have previously had a cesarean.

▲ Ask your caregiver whether having an epidural might increase your cesarean risk. Early administration of some types of epidurals has been associated with higher cesarean, vacuum, and forceps rates.

▲ Ask whether your caregiver would try to turn a baby who is in breech position (see page 103) after 37 weeks of pregnancy, or would consider letting you deliver a breech baby vaginally *and* could assure that a birth attendant experienced in vaginal breeches will be available at delivery.

▲ Take a childbirth class to learn about obstetric interventions and effective non-drug methods of coping with labor pain.

▲ Plan to use natural methods to encourage labor progress, such as walking during labor and squatting for pushing.

▲ Use electronic fetal monitoring only intermittently, or request telemetry monitoring so you can stay upright and mobile during labor.

▲ Bring a trained labor companion (see page 151) to the hospital with you.

▲ Request a second opinion if your caregiver recommends a nonemergency cesarean or any cesarean that seems questionable to you.

IF YOU NEED A CESAREAN   Of course, not every cesarean should be prevented. This operation has saved the lives of many mothers and babies. Although most women don't anticipate a surgical birth, about one out of seven first-time mothers ends up with one. So it's a good idea to learn about the procedure during pregnancy and to express any preferences you may have about your care.

Today most cesareans are performed under regional anesthesia, such as epidural (see page 150) or spinal block, both of which numb the mother from the nipples down but leave her awake for the birth. If a cesarean is done in an emergency, a mother may require general anesthesia, which quickly puts her to sleep before surgery begins.

The surgical procedure takes an hour or so. The baby is born within about ten minutes after the anesthesia takes effect. Stitching up takes at least 30 minutes.

A cesarean proceeds this way: The mother's abdomen may be shaved and is washed, and a catheter (drainage tube) is put into her bladder. An intravenous needle is inserted into her wrist to provide her with fluids and any necessary medications. Once she is numb, the doctor makes an incision in her abdomen. Except in an emergency, or if an obstetrical reason dictates the less common vertical cut, the doctor makes a small, horizontal "bikini" cut, just above the pubic bone. Like the abdominal incision, the uterine cut can also be horizontal or vertical. A vertical uterine incision, which usually dictates future cesareans, may be needed to save time in an emergency, or because of the position of the baby or placenta. The doctor next opens the amniotic sac and lifts out the baby. If the mother is awake during the birth she usually feels some tugging, pulling, or pressure. The doctor then removes the placenta and closes the incisions in the uterus and abdomen.

To make your cesarean, anticipated or not, the best birth possible, ask your medical caregiver if you can:

▲ use an epidural or spinal block rather than general anesthesia, if possible, so you can be awake to greet your baby.

▲ have your partner stay with you in the operating room while your baby is born.

▲ hear the doctor's running account of the birth.

▲ watch or videotape the delivery.

▲ choose whether or not you would like pre-operative or post-operative medications.

▲ keep one arm free to touch your baby after the birth.

▲ hold and nurse your baby in the recovery room while the anesthetic is still in effect.

▲ have **transcutaneous electric nerve stimulation (TENS)** electrodes applied on either side of your incision right after delivery so you will need less narcotic medication in the early postpartum period; and

▲ get a narcotic injected into your spinal or epidural space after the birth. This kind of pain relief lasts about 24 hours and doesn't interfere with breastfeeding or walking, cause constipation, or make you feel nauseated. At hospitals where this option is unavailable, mothers are given oral or intravenous pain killers.

Also ask about the options for post-cesarean recuperation listed on page 187.

VBAC   Once a cesarean, *not* always a cesarean. Routine repeat cesareans became the rule in the early 1900s, when the then-rare surgery was typically performed with a lengthwise cut through the uterus. This vertical uterine incision threatened rupture during subsequent labors. For decades afterward the rule held firm, even though obstetricians began to perform most cesareans with low, horizontal incisions. In fact, these horizontal cervical incisions heal strongly enough to make an attempted vaginal birth after cesarean (VBAC) as safe as or even safer than a repeat cesarean for many mothers.

The VBAC rate rose from 2 percent in 1975 to 28 percent in 1996 before falling to 12.6 percent in 2002. Many women can undergo VBAC safely, but the risks of labor must be weighed against the risks of a major operative procedure. Your decision will be based on many factors, including your preference and that of your caregiver and the facility you have chosen for delivery.

If you have had a cesarean, are you a good candidate for a VBAC? Probably. You need—

▲ a normal-sized pelvis;
▲ a horizontal uterine incision (your abdominal incision does not matter);
▲ a pregnancy with just one baby, in a head-first position; and
▲ a positive and encouraging caregiver.

A VBAC carries some risks, as does every birth, including a routine repeat cesarean. The main risk of VBAC is rupture of the uterine scar, which happens in fewer than 1 percent of cases in which the uterine incision is horizontal. If rupture occurs, an emergency cesarean may be necessary.

Be sure your caregiver presents a balanced view of the risks and benefits as they apply to you. Then form a reasonable birth plan, be sure your caregiver and birth partner support it, and keep your plan flexible enough to avoid subjecting yourself and your baby to unnecessary dangers. Like any obstetric facility, the hospital where you plan to have your VBAC should be prepared to perform an emergency cesarean within 30 minutes. Your hospital should also provide electronic fetal monitoring (see page 136) and a fully equipped blood bank. Although many women have successful VBACs at home, the small (approximately .5 percent) risk of uterine rupture with VBAC probably makes the hospital a safer place for these births.

What if you end up needing another cesarean after attempting a VBAC? You have a right to feel disappointed, but take some consolation in the fact that your efforts have done your baby a favor. Babies who experience at least some labor have fewer breathing problems at birth. And many mothers feel better just for having attempted a vaginal birth.

Pain Relief in Labor

Birth is thrilling, but having a baby usually hurts—a lot. Labor hurts for several good reasons. For one thing, hours of effort tire your hard-working uterus, which must contract mightily to expel the baby. In addition, these strong contractions cause your cervix to expand, which you may feel as increasingly intense cramping, pressure, or stretching. The baby's passage down and out can put uncomfortable pressure on your back, bladder, and bowel. And your vagina must stretch to accommodate the baby's passage. Ouch.

At the end of nine months, however, your body is perfectly ready to give birth. And, no matter how much any one contraction hurts, you usually get a rest before the next one starts. Given a normal labor, your main task is to go along with the process.

One aspect of labor you *can* control is how you cope with the pain, including the decision of whether or not to use medication. Unless you're planning to give birth at home or in a birth center, you can put off making a final decision about medication until labor is underway. But think and talk about the subject now. If you prefer to avoid medication, for example, your helpers should support you instead of pressuring you to get an epidural. If you lean toward medication, find out what your hospital offers; not every hospital provides every form of pain relief. In addition, tell your caregiver if you've ever had a negative reaction to any drugs, such as the anesthetics your dentist uses.

NON-DRUG METHODS   If you opt not to use drugs for labor, don't let anyone put down your preference by calling you a martyr. Relying on your own strength to meet the challenge of labor can give you a great sense of accomplishment, like successfully completing a marathon.

What if your birth partner is unenthusiastic about your goal? Seek support and counseling from your childbirth educator, or consider hiring a supportive labor companion (see page 151). Your birth attendants, including your caregiver and nurse, should back up your choice but promise to support you if circumstances dictate a change of plans.

Any drug you take during labor has potential side effects on your baby, you, and your labor. Since non-drug methods have few side effects, always consider them first for coping with labor pain. Even if you're pretty sure you want to use pain medication, there's another good reason to learn some natural methods of pain relief. To avoid interfering with the progress of your labor, your caregivers will likely offer painkillers only after your labor is well under way. So most mothers need to use non-drug methods for at least part of labor.

Try these non-drug methods to ease labor pain:

▲ Relax your muscles.

▲ Breathe calmly during and between your contractions.

▲ Focus on something soothing, such as a picture, mental image, or recorded musical tape.

▲ If labor is slow, stay upright and walk as long as you can to promote its progress.

▲ When you need to rest, experiment to find a comfortable position. Avoid lying on your back; instead, try standing, kneeling, leaning, side-lying, squatting, sitting, or the all-fours position (see pages 128 to 130).

▲ Drink juice, tea, or bouillon.

▲ Avoid uncomfortable interventions such as an enema or IV, if possible.

▲ Take a warm bath or shower.

▲ Consider spending your labor in warm water; birth tubs are available at some birthing centers and hospitals and can be rented for a home birth.

▲ Use ice compresses, hot packs, or pressure for back pain (see page 176).

▲ Have a supportive partner or partners with you.

▲ Ask for a back rub or a hand or foot massage.

▲ Ask your labor nurse for other suggestions; for example, some hospitals provide large inflated balls for comfort and support in labor.

Any good childbirth class (see page 123) should teach a variety of natural techniques for managing pain. Practicing these techniques can boost your confidence, which is more important than you might think. Women who expect patterned breathing and relaxation to help during labor find these techniques much more helpful than do doubters.

Non-drug methods can offer enough relief for a normal labor. Should your labor prove harder, the tips listed above can help you put off medication or reduce the amount you'll need.

MEDICATION Despite what you may have heard, no drug can guarantee a pain-free labor without some drawbacks. For example, taking medication will usually keep you from walking, an activity that speeds labor and eases pain. If medication slows your progress, you may need Pitocin (see page 138), forceps, or a cesarean. Each of these interventions involves further risks. Finally, drugs may affect your baby.

On the plus side, medications usually do decrease pain. In addition they can sometimes promote progress by helping the mother relax. Medication can also aid a complicated delivery.

Try to familiarize yourself with the benefits and risks of some commonly used medications before you go into labor. Find out what specific medications can do for you and what they might do to you, your labor, and your baby. Then you'll be able to make an informed decision during labor. If you choose medication, you will probably be offered narcotics or an epidural block.

Narcotics Your labor nurse or prenatal caregiver may give narcotics such as Demerol, Stadol, Dilaudid, Fentanyl, or Nubain in a shot, through your IV, or by both methods in a divided dose, after your cervix has dilated to about 4 centimeters. Moderate pain relief, often described as "taking the edge off," lasts for two to four hours, when the dosage can be repeated. Possible side effects from narcotics include a lowering of your blood pressure, which could make you feel ill and threaten your baby's well-being. Narcotics could also make you experience nausea, vomiting, dizziness, confusion, dry mouth, and breathing problems. Occasionally a tranquilizer such as Phenergan is given along with the narcotic to decrease nausea.

Given too close to birth, narcotics can block a baby's first breathing efforts, so you probably won't get a first or repeat dose after you are dilated to about 8 centimeters. If narcotics do cause a breathing delay, your baby may be given a shot of a narcotic antagonist such as Narcan, which immediately reverses this temporary problem.

Epidural   In contrast to narcotics, an epidural relieves pain effectively without affecting the mind. At some hospitals, epidurals have become so popular that they are practically routine.

This is how an epidural is given: An anesthesiologist inserts a tiny, flexible catheter into the mother's back, just outside the dura, or spinal membrane. Typically, a combination of anesthetic and narcotic drugs flows through the catheter into the epidural space. Relief arrives about ten minutes after the drugs are administered. Since she will be somewhat numbed below the waist, the mother must usually remain in bed afterward. But a few hospitals currently offer the option of a "walking epidural," which combines an epidural anesthetic with the spinal administration of narcotics to allow more movement during labor and pushing.

An epidural can offer excellent pain relief for labor, though the mother may also need a local anesthetic for the repair of an episiotomy or a tear. Administered to anesthetize more of the body, an epidural can also be used for a cesarean delivery.

Some research has linked epidurals during labor to higher rates of cesarean and assisted deliveries, such as forceps births. Other research finds epidurals do not make cesareans more likely. But an epidural can retard labor. Should your epidural slow the process, intravenous Pitocin will probably be able to speed it up again. If the epidural interferes with your pushing efforts, the IV infusion can be slowed or stopped. These measures will allow natural feeling to return.

Though epidurals typically work well, they do have drawbacks. Some women experience incomplete numbness. Also, once or twice in 100 epidurals, the spinal membrane is accidentally punctured, leading to a nasty but treatable "spinal headache." There are often other maternal side effects, such as lowered blood pressure, itching, and urinary retention, although these can be minimized with attentive medical care.

Does an epidural affect the baby? Some experts believe epidurals cause temporary glitches with nursing by impairing a baby's alertness and early sucking efforts. To avoid these problems, try to nurse your baby as soon after birth as possible, be patient, and keep trying.

Birth Helpers

Labor is one time in life when you definitely need a friend. Most women enlist the help of a birth partner. In addition, some women arrange for an extra helper, often called a doula, to provide extra support and encouragement. Today many hospitals also welcome the baby's siblings at the birth.

YOUR BIRTH PARTNER Being together for labor and birth can strengthen the special bond between a couple. Your birth partner—probably your husband or mate, but perhaps a close friend or relative—can help you physically and emotionally. He can provide physical support by massaging your tense shoulders or sore back, offering his hand to clutch, mopping your brow with a cool washcloth, feeding you ice chips, holding your hand as you stroll the halls, reminding you to breathe and relax, and perhaps supporting you as you push. Emotional support might include calming your fears, encouraging you, and lavishly praising your efforts.

Plan to attend childbirth classes (see page 123) with your birth partner. There you'll both learn how to work together during labor.

SHOULD YOU BRING A DOULA? If you want to keep your child's birth as private as possible, you may want your partner to be your sole labor companion. But if you have no partner, if your partner would not make the best labor helper, or if he may be unavailable when labor starts, you may want the additional support of an experienced labor companion.

An extra labor companion—usually a woman—is often called by the Greek name *doula* to indicate her main task: mothering the mother. Women who assist mothers at home after birth are also called doulas. During labor, a doula can help you cope with labor, relieve and support your birth partner, and explain your needs to the hospital staff. This birth companion may also help the over-worked nursing staff to give you one-on-one care during labor. Some doulas are private-duty nurses, who examine women at home and listen to the baby's heart tones. But even a doula who offers nothing more than basic physical and emotional support offers a lot. Research suggests that the presence of a doula short-ens labor, and cuts the rate of fetal distress, Pitocin, epidural, anesthesia, forceps use, and cesareans.

If you opt to use a doula, you may choose a close friend or rel-ative with an interest in childbirth. The most important qualifica-tion is that your doula be loving and nonjudgmental. Ask yourself if you will feel good having this person around when you feel vulnerable.

Or you may choose to hire a professional doula (see "Re-sources"). Be sure to confirm with your caregiver that your doula will be welcome at the hospital. Aside from your personal comfort with a prospective doula, consider her experience with and atti-tudes about birth. Ask what services are included in her fee, when she will be available and who will substitute for her when she's not, and what relationship she has with your hospital. You may also want to check references from satisfied clients.

SIBLINGS   Parents disagree on whether children should be pres-ent at birth. So do experts. Some argue that the sights and sounds of birth are disturbing to children. Others feel that, with advance planning, birth can be a joyous family event.

At home births siblings are normally present and easily accommodated, since their beds and toys are close by. Most birth centers welcome siblings, too. Some hospitals, however, don't. If you'd like your older children to accompany you to the hospital for the birth, and if they want to be there, find out whether your hospital and your caregiver will allow this choice.

It's as important for your child to be prepared for birth as it is for you and your partner to take childbirth classes. Most hospitals that permit siblings to be present for the birth offer a special class just for them. In such a class your child can learn about what hap-pens during labor, how he can help by offering ice chips or hold-ing your hand, and how a newborn looks and acts.

Be sure that attending the birth is something your child wants to do for himself, not for you. At some point before or during labor your child may decide that he doesn't want to stay around for the birth. Let him make that decision.

Your Birth Plan

In a hospital delivery, much of your care may be given by nurses and resident or "house" physicians you've never seen before. A written birth plan is one way to communicate about what you prefer. A birth plan shouldn't be a list of your demands, but a product of cooperation between you and your caregiver. Because no one can script birth in advance, the language you use in your plan should show flexibility. Phrases like "we prefer," "if conditions permit," and "if possible" let doctors and nurses know you're allowing for the unpredictability of labor.

You needn't include every aspect of birth in your plan. If you know, for example, that your birth attendant and hospital usually honor certain of your choices, simply skip those. But be sure to include all items that differ from the standard treatment. Remember to plan for a complicated or cesarean delivery as well as for your ideal delivery. In fact, in difficult deliveries it's especially important to have some say in your medical care.

In your birth plan, you may want to ask for—

▲ freedom to change positions and walk during labor;

▲ monitoring by stethoscope, Doppler, or radio telemetry instead of standard electronic fetal monitoring;

▲ no routine amniotomy;

▲ no routine episiotomy;

▲ permission to eat, or drink at least, instead of having an IV;

▲ certain medications or other pain relief methods;

▲ permission to have extra partners present during labor and birth;

▲ regional rather than general anesthesia if you need a cesarean, and your partner's presence in the operating room;

▲ rooming in, or having the baby brought to you whenever she cries;

▲ breastfeeding help; and

▲ early release from the hospital, or the longest stay your medical plan will allow.

After you and your caregiver agree on your birth plan, ask that it be inserted into your prenatal record or attached to it. Be sure to save your own copy to bring to the hospital. And keep in mind that, although you've communicated your preferences, you can always change your mind after labor begins.

Because you'll need to give your primary attention to labor and birth, plan to bring along an extra companion to be responsible for each child. This companion should be prepared to explain what is happening or to take your child out for a break if necessary. You and your partner should also feel free to change your minds and have your child escorted out if labor proves unexpectedly difficult.

With appropriate support and education, birth can be a wonderful shared family experience. Most medical professionals with experience in sibling-attended births give a hearty thumbs up to parents who want to try it. But even though some experts still maintain that a sibling's place is *not* in the birthing room, today almost all hospitals and birthing centers enthusiastically encourage sibling visits after the birth to see their mother and greet the new baby.

Baby-care Options

Some of your choices for childbirth concern the newborn baby. Pregnancy is a good time to find out about what happens in a baby's first hours, about cord-blood banking, and about circumcision. You'll probably also want to give some thought to your baby's name (see page 156).

Your Baby's First Hours

Contrary to popular opinion, **bonding**—the development of an emotional attachment between mother and newborn—doesn't happen automatically in the moment when the baby is placed on the mother's chest at birth. Instead, bonding is a gradual process of getting to know and love a newborn. Families who miss spending time together in the birthing room, for a variety of reasons (cesarean birth, a sick newborn, an exhausted mother) will get plenty of chances to become bonded in the coming days and weeks.

Think of the first hour or two after birth not as a critical period but as a great opportunity. This period is an ideal time for falling in love, because right after birth newborns are wide awake and bright-eyed. Your baby can see well at a distance of about 8 to 12 inches, and will gaze right into your eyes if the light is dimmed. And your newborn can keep warm when nestled skin to skin with you. In fact, recent research suggests that, if placed on her mother's abdomen, a newborn baby can instinctively creep up to find the nipple and begin nursing without any help at all.

Plan to take advantage of this exciting period by asking in advance to lift your baby up yourself or to hold her immediately after birth as long as you are both in good condition. Your caregiver can easily delay the eye treatment (see page 192) that will temporarily cloud your baby's vision, as well as weighing, measuring, footprinting, and wiping. If you plan to nurse, the first hour or two is an ideal time to start (see page 193).

Cord-blood Banking

After a baby is born in a hospital, her umbilical cord blood is typically thrown away along with the placenta. But, like bone marrow, umbilical cord blood is rich in stem cells. These unspecialized blood cells can produce other kinds of blood cells, making them a precious resource to treat blood and immune disorders. Stem cells may also be able to cure some cancers.

Donated bone marrow supplies most current medical needs for stem cells. But harvesting stem cells from bone marrow requires painful surgery for the donor. In contrast, stem cells from cord blood can be collected painlessly from the umbilical cord immediately after birth. In addition, because cord blood stem cells are immature, they pose a smaller risk of rejection than do stem cells harvested from the bone marrow of an adult donor. A little bit of cord blood goes a long way, too; cord blood contains almost ten times as many stem cells as does the same weight of bone marrow.

You can have your baby's cord blood collected and stored for your own family's use, or you can donate it to a public cord-blood bank in the way you might donate your own blood. In the first case, you would pay for storage and maintenance. In 2004, initial collection fees ranged from $595 to $1,740, and maintenance fees were about $100 each year. You might consider this cost worthwhile if you have a family history of genetic disease such as severe anemia, an immune disorder, or any of certain cancers. Without such risk factors, the chances are about one in ten thousand that a member of your family will ever need a stem cell transplantation.

If you choose to donate your baby's cord blood, a public cord-blood bank will foot the bill for processing and storing the donation. But the bank will require you to undergo tests before the birth for diseases such as hepatitis and HIV and to complete a

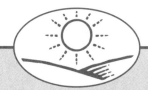

Name That Baby

In the hospital, you'll be asked your baby's name for the birth certificate, which must usually be filed within several days of birth. Some parents need to see their babies before deciding, but most parents choose names beforehand.

If you decide to test some of your possible choices on family and friends, grow a thick skin. People are much likelier to let you know what they really think of your choices before the baby is born than they will if you hold off your announcement until afterward.

Can't make up your mind, or change your mind after the birth certificate is filed? It's your responsibility to call the appropriate agency—clerk of court, county recorder, or auditor—to make additions or changes.

Classics like Michael, Matthew, Elizabeth, and Catherine remain popular generation after generation. But some names—especially girls'—cycle in and out of vogue. If you want to avoid having yours be one of five children in the classroom with the same trendy name, read the newspaper birth announcements, and ask other women in your childbirth class what names they're thinking of.

Looking for an unusual name for your baby? You're in luck, because books on baby naming fill shelves in the library and bookstore. Experts advise parents playing the baby-name game to keep a few pointers in mind:

▲ Your child will have this name for a long time. Ask yourself: Will it suit a baby? A child? A young adult? A rock guitarist? A Supreme Court justice? A grandparent?
▲ Try to avoid names that are hard to pronounce or spell.
▲ Find first and middle names that sound good with your baby's last name.
▲ Consider whether the initials will make an embarrassing monogram, like B.O. or N.U.T.
▲ Don't choose a name with a nickname you dislike; your child's friends will be bound to use it.

health questionnaire. Ask your caregiver how to make arrangements with a public cord-blood bank at least two months before your due date. These simple actions could save someone's life.

Circumcision

If your new baby is a boy, you'll need to decide whether to have him circumcised. Shortly before you go home from the hospital, a physician can perform this minor operation, which severs the foreskin of the baby's penis. Or you may wait for several days or weeks before having the circumcision performed in the doctor's office. Jewish ritual circumcision is typically performed at home on the eighth day after birth by a skilled professional called a *mohel.*

Parents who opt for non-ritual circumcision typically choose the surgery not for medical benefits but for social reasons. For example, parents may want their newborn son to look like his circumcised father, older brother, or future locker room buddies. Currently about 61 percent of boys born in the United States are circumcised. The rate differs by region, however: In 1999, 81 percent of boys in the Midwest were circumcised, compared to only 37 percent of boys in the West. In the Northeast and South, circumcision rates were 65 and 64 percent, respectively.

Some parents choose the operation because of assumptions about cleanliness. In fact, teaching an uncircumcised boy to keep his penis clean is about as challenging as teaching him to wash behind his ears: difficult but doable.

Medical experts neither recommend nor discourage circumcision. In 1999, the American Academy of Pediatrics Task Force on Circumcision said the procedure's medical advantages—lower incidences of urinary tract infections in childhood and a very rare form of cancer in adulthood—were insufficient to recommend routine circumcision. Parents must weigh the possible advantages against the pain of the operation and the small possibility of complications, including bleeding, injury, and infection.

The American Academy of Pediatrics recommends topical or injected local anesthesia that safely reduces the pain of circumcision. If you choose a medical circumcision, ask whether your caregiver uses such medication. And if your infant is sick or premature, consider delaying the surgery for days or weeks until he is stronger.

Postpartum Options

Whether the first weeks with your baby are idyllic or exhausting may depend on your advance preparations. Choose your baby's doctor, line up home help, and prepare your house and car for your baby's arrival.

Choosing a Baby Doctor

If your health plan gives you a choice of baby doctors, find the one you feel most comfortable with. Because it's easier to visit doctors when you aren't toting a newborn baby and a diaper bag, try to

Baby Doctors You might ask a prospective baby doctor some of these questions:

Are you certified or eligible for certification by the American Board of Pediatrics or the American Board of Family Practice?

Do you practice solo or in a group?

Will you examine my baby right after the birth? Can I observe this examination?

How soon will you see my baby after we go home from the hospital?

How often will routine visits be scheduled?

What happens at a checkup?

What are your hours and fees?

Which hospital would you admit my baby to if the baby needed to be hospitalized?

How do you handle emergency calls? Nonemergency calls?

How do you encourage breastfeeding?

Do you recommend circumcision? Why or why not?

You might also ask about day care, pacifiers, weaning, vegetarianism, and sleeping with the baby.

interview prospective doctors for your baby before you give birth. Get recommendations from friends or relatives with young children or from your birth attendant. Ask these people what they like about the doctor they recommend.

Most pediatricians and family practitioners welcome expectant parents. But be sure to ask in advance whether you will be charged for their time.

Lining Up Home Help

Expect to need some assistance after you get home. Having your partner stay home from work for a week or more after you return home can help a lot. Also, ask friends and relatives to pitch in. You can spread out your help by limiting these visitors to one or two at a time.

Your helpers' role should be to do the housework or watch older children while you and your husband attend to the baby and try to grab some rest. A responsible neighborhood teenager may also be able to take on some of these tasks.

Of course, you'll need extra time and pampering to recuperate from a cesarean or a difficult vaginal birth. In such a case you may want to consider hiring a professional. In many cities, postpartum doula services include anything from meal preparation to hands-on breastfeeding assistance. Costs vary by location, but usually range from $15 to about $30 per hour, with a minimum of several hours per day. The National Association of Postpartum Care Services, which certifies postpartum doulas, requires that they be trained in breastfeeding, infant care and CPR, and postpartum recovery care (see "Resources").

Home Help When you interview someone for postpartum help, you may want to ask these questions:

What is your training and experience?

Are you certified or licensed?

Can I call some of the women you've worked for recently?

What is your philosophy of baby care?

Buying a Car Seat

To transport your baby home safely you'll need a car seat that complies with current federal standards. You can choose an infant-only seat, which allows your infant to recline and will accommodate her until she weighs 20 pounds; or a convertible seat, which accommodates babies and toddlers weighing up to 40 pounds.

You needn't spend extra money on a car seat that doubles as an infant carrier. At home, your baby is better off in your arms, supported against your body in a pouch or sling, sitting in a bouncer set, or lying on a blanket on the floor.

Purchase a new car seat, if you can, because a used one may be damaged or missing parts or instructions. If you opt for a used car seat, make sure that it—

▲ is less than six years old,
▲ has a label advertising conformity with the Federal Motor Vehicle Safety standards,
▲ includes instructions, and
▲ has never been in a crash.

Learn how to install the car seat before you go to the hospital or birth center. To do this, you may need to check your vehicle owner's manual.

Getting Your Other Baby Gear

You can purchase everything else you need after you bring your baby home. Or you may want to begin collecting some of these items before you give birth:

▲ A crib or bassinet, along with a firm mattress, bumper guards, sheets, waterproof pads, and blanket. Cribs manufactured after 1985 boast essential safety features— slats less than $2\frac{3}{8}$ inches apart and no leaded paint or varnish.
▲ Four to six receiving blankets—small, lightweight blankets for swaddling (snugly wrapping) your newborn.
▲ A weekly supply of about 70 disposable or 90 cloth diapers, as well as several pairs of waterproof pants or diaper covers; diaper pins, if needed; and a diaper pail if you plan to use cloth diapers. If you choose disposable diapers, you may want to purchase some cloth diapers

to use for burp cloths. Keep in mind that disposable diapers come in different sizes and that your baby will grow. In cities and suburbs, you may have the option of a diaper service to deliver clean diapers each week.

▲ If you're planning to bottle-feed, two 4-ounce bottles with nipples, eight 8-ounce bottles with nipples, several nipple rings and nipple covers, a bottle and nipple brush, and a holder for washing nipples and nipple rings in your dishwasher. If you're planning to breastfeed, purchase at least one bottle for emergency use.

▲ Washcloths and hooded towels.

▲ Six to ten undershirts (your baby may prefer the kind that snap in front).

▲ Four to six gowns (optional).

▲ Four to six "onesies," or body suits.

▲ Four to six "stretchies," or footed coveralls.

▲ Blanket sleepers, sweaters, hat, and snowsuit for cold weather; a sunbonnet for warm weather.

▲ Two to four pairs of socks or booties.

▲ Baby soap and shampoo.

▲ Rubbing alcohol and cotton balls for umbilical stump care.

▲ Cornstarch-based baby powder.

▲ Blunt-tipped scissors for cutting nails.

▲ A rectal thermometer and K-Y or another water-soluble lubricating jelly. For infants over six months, ear thermometers are reliable and easier to use, but they are also costly.

▲ Liquid acetaminophen pain reliever.

▲ Bulb syringe for clearing a stuffy nose.

You may also want to buy, borrow, or beg for some of these other helpful items:

▲ a cloth carrier to snuggle your baby close to your heart while you walk,

▲ a stroller,

▲ a baby monitor so you can hear the baby when you're sleeping or working in another room,

▲ a bouncing infant seat,

▲ a swing, and

▲ a cool-mist humidifier to ease the baby's breathing during a cold.

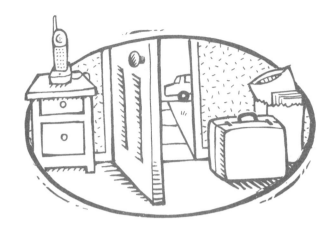

CHAPTER 8

A Labor of Love

After months of waiting, your baby is finally ready to be born. Laboring to deliver her may take several days or may speed by in an intense hour or two. First labors average about 12 to 14 hours, and subsequent labors approximately 8 hours.

What Happens During Labor?

During labor, involuntary contractions pull up your cervix (the neck-like bottom portion of your uterus) and open it around your baby's head. Once your cervix is completely effaced (thinned out) and dilated (opened up) labor contractions press your baby's head into the vagina, or birth canal. Then you add conscious effort to the pushing action of the uterus, giving birth to your baby. After birth, contractions expel your placenta and help shrink your uterus back down to its original size.

You're likely to hear these terms to describe your body's readiness for labor and the progress of your labor:

▲ **Effacement:** the thinning or drawing up of the cervix with the Braxton-Hicks contractions or the earliest labor

Effacement

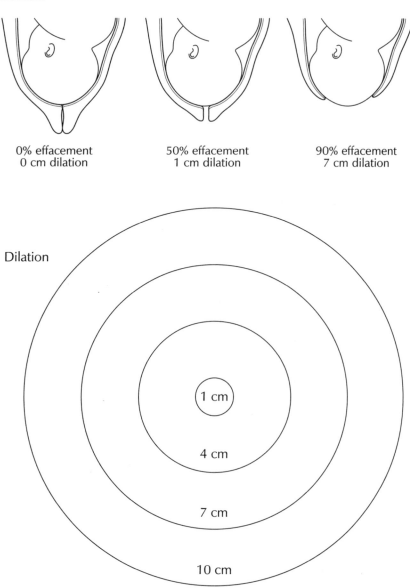

0% effacement 0 cm dilation	50% effacement 1 cm dilation	90% effacement 7 cm dilation

Dilation

1 cm

4 cm

7 cm

10 cm

contractions. A vaginal exam can estimate the amount of effacement from 0 percent, when the cervix is long and thick, to 100 percent, when it is completely thinned out and taken up into the rest of the uterus.

▲ **Dilation or dilatation:** the opening of the cervix, a process that speeds up after the cervix has effaced, or thinned out. With later babies, the cervix typically begins to dilate even before it effaces. In a vaginal examination, a caregiver can estimate your dilation from undilated or one fingertip dilated (about 1 to 2 centimeters, as big as a Cheerio) to completely dilated (about 10 centimeters, the size of a large navel orange).

▲ **Station:** the level of the baby's descent. When the top of your baby's head—the part that usually comes out first—reaches a landmark called the ischial spines (the bones that support you when you sit), your baby's head is said to be at station 0, or engaged. Engagement means the baby will almost certainly fit through the mother's pelvis.

Although first babies tend to engage at some time during the month before delivery, later babies typically engage only after labor begins. Station numbers range from –4 to +4; the numbers represent centimeters. A baby who is at –4, or far from being engaged, may be termed "floating." Station –1 means the head is 1 centimeter from being engaged, station +1 means the head is 1 centimeter past being engaged, and so on. At station +4, the baby's head has come through the birth canal.

Not Too Early, Not Too Late

Dated from a woman's last menstrual period, pregnancy usually lasts between 37 and 42 weeks. A baby born well before the due date may have problems eating, breathing, and keeping warm. When pregnancy lasts too long, an aging placenta may fail to nourish the baby, amniotic fluid may decrease, and the baby may become stressed.

PRETERM LABOR   Labor that begins before 37 weeks can sometimes be delayed with medication, giving a baby a stronger start. Although it's normal to feel uterine contractions in late pregnancy (see page 84), when they come as often as four in an hour they may cause your cervix to dilate too soon. The following symptoms can signify labor contractions:

▲ feelings of tightening in the abdomen,
▲ a menstrual-type cramping sensation in the groin,

▲ a low, dull backache that doesn't go away even when you change position,

▲ pressure in the pelvis or thighs,

▲ intestinal cramping or loose stools, and

Leaking water may mean your bag of waters has ruptured. If this happens, call your caregiver.

If you think you may be in preterm labor, take these steps:

▲ Stop doing whatever you were doing when contractions began.

▲ Lie down on your left side.

▲ Drink two to three glasses of water.

▲ If you continue to have four or more contractions per hour, call your caregiver. You'll probably need to go to the hospital to be examined.

▲ If your symptoms disappear, return to light activity, but be sure to let your caregiver know what happened.

▲ Should symptoms return, call your caregiver immediately.

To help determine the appropriate treatment, your caregiver may suggest a procedure called a **fetal fibronectin test,** in which a sample of fluid is taken from the vagina. Finding the protein fetal fibronectin in this smear means that the fetal sac may be beginning to detach from the uterus and that premature labor will probably recur.

You will also be examined internally to see whether your cervix has begun to dilate. Depending on when your baby is due and how much your cervix has opened, you may be given medication to stop the contractions, and you may need to spend the next few days or weeks on bed rest (see page 119). If your baby is coming more than three weeks early, you may also have an amniocentesis (see page 39) to check your baby's lung maturity. The results can suggest whether your labor should be delayed if possible, or whether labor can safely be allowed to continue. The amniocentesis can also show whether you should receive corticosteroid medication. In certain situations, corticosteroids given to a mother can help her baby's lungs mature and protect the newborn's fragile brain from the bleeding that sometimes occurs in premies.

DELAYED LABOR Most pregnancies that exceed 41 or even 42 weeks pose no problem to the baby. Some babies simply require a little extra growing time. But occasionally when labor fails to begin on time, an aging placenta can deprive a baby of needed nourishment. If you go more than a week beyond your due date, you may undergo tests to determine whether or not it is safe to continue your pregnancy. You may be asked to take some or all of these tests:

- ▲ a nonstress test (see page 40),
- ▲ a contraction stress test (see page 40),
- ▲ a biophysical profile (see page 42) or ultrasound exam, and
- ▲ a determination of amniotic fluid volume (see page 42).

If your labor must be induced, ask which methods are safest and most effective, because long or painful contractions could stress your baby. Discuss with your caregiver the benefits and drawbacks of both medical induction and these home methods:

- ▲ **Castor oil, an enema, or both:** Bowel action produces prostaglandins that can stimulate cervical change and contractions.
- ▲ **Genital stimulation:** Especially if it leads to orgasm, sex can cause contractions. But avoid inserting anything into your vagina if your membranes have ruptured.
- ▲ **Nipple stimulation:** Stroking or rolling your nipples can cause contractions. Stimulate one nipple at a time, take frequent breaks, and stop if you have a contraction that lasts for 45 seconds or more.
- ▲ **Herbal teas:** Red raspberry leaf tea (available at any health-food store) has long been touted as a labor enhancer. Pour 1 pint of boiling water over 1 ounce of raspberry leaves, cover, and steep the leaves for half an hour. Then strain the tea and drink it hot. If your caregiver agrees, you could take an insulated bottle of raspberry leaf tea to the hospital with you.

  Herbalists and homeopathic physicians also sometimes recommend caulophyllum, or blue cohosh, to promote stronger contractions. But this herb can also increase blood pressure and irritate the mucous membranes. Before using blue cohosh or other herbal remedies during labor, check with a knowledgeable person.

If you need an induction, your caregiver may use one or more of the following medical methods:

- ▲ **Stripping the membranes:** If your cervix is dilated enough, your caregiver can insert a finger and gently separate the bottom portion of the membranes from the uterus. This sometimes starts labor.
- ▲ **Prostaglandin:** Used in the form of a gel or vaginal or oral tablet, prostaglandin softens the cervix, making it much more likely to dilate easily when Pitocin is given (see page 138).
- ▲ **Laminaria or catheter:** Laminaria tents are seaweed or synthetic strips that, when placed in the wet environment of the birth canal, stretch and dilate the cervix. Some hospitals instead use catheters, or rubber tubes, with expandable balloons to stretch the cervical opening. Because inserting anything into the birth canal slightly raises the risk of infection, these devices are used only when a firm decision has been made to speed the delivery.
- ▲ **Pitocin:** Administration of this synthetic form of the hormone oxytocin is the most commonly used method to induce labor. Given intravenously so that the dose can be very carefully controlled, Pitocin works most effectively on a soft cervix that has already begun to dilate (see pages 164 and 138).
- ▲ **Rupture of membranes:** If your membranes don't break naturally after labor has begun, your caregiver may painlessly rupture them with a long hook. Whether natural or artificial, membrane rupture can speed up labor (see "Amniotomy," page 139).

Getting Ready for Labor

You may experience one or more of these signs in the weeks and days before you give birth. Though you needn't call your caregiver to report any of these signs, noticing them should definitely encourage you. Your pregnancy is almost over.

- ▲ **Engagement** (see page 164): Your baby drops down to nestle deep within your pelvis. This change will offer you some relief from any breathlessness you've experienced, but you may begin to experience increasing heaviness in your pelvis and legs.

▲ **Increased vaginal discharge:** This mucus discharge may be tinged pink or brown (see "Bloody Show," below).

▲ **Backache:** If back pains come and go frequently, and regularly, you may be experiencing contractions (see page 169).

▲ **Weight loss:** You may lose a pound or two, thanks to the hormonal changes that precede labor.

▲ **Soft, frequent stools:** Early labor can cause intestinal movement, prompting the production of prostaglandins that soften the cervix and make it more likely to dilate.

▲ **A burst of energy:** Many women report feeling a "nesting urge" that makes them want to clean house, move furniture, or fill their freezer with meals for after the baby comes. Indulge this happy urge, but save some energy for labor.

▲ **Cervical changes:** In a vaginal examination, your caregiver might notice that your cervix has begun to soften, efface (see page 162), or dilate (see page 164).

Signs of Labor

Any of the following signs means that your labor will probably begin soon or that it has already started.

BLOODY SHOW   As your cervix begins to thin and open, blood from the many tiny cervical blood vessels often mixes with the plug of mucus that lines the opening of the cervix. The blood gives this so-called mucus plug a pinkish color. The mucus plug may come out in the toilet or it may show up on your underpants. Seeing the bloody show usually means that your labor will begin within the next day or two. But because your cervix can begin to dilate a few weeks before labor begins, a bloody show may precede labor by as long as 20 days. Too, because the plug may not contain blood, many women never even notice it. **Remember that a continuous flow of bright red bleeding should be reported to your caregiver immediately.** A small amount of brown or red blood may be harmless spotting from the cervix following intercourse or a vaginal exam. But the appearance of bright red blood could signify a problem with your placenta, such as its separation from the uterus (placental abruption) or its blockage of the cervix (placenta previa).

RUPTURE OF THE MEMBRANES   A sudden gush or a more typical slow trickle of fluid from your vagina means that your bag of waters has sprung a leak. Your bag of waters may break before contractions begin or at any time during labor. How can you tell whether you are losing amniotic fluid or urine? Doing your Kegels (see page 63) should stop the flow of urine, but amniotic fluid will continue to trickle out despite your efforts to stop it. So empty your bladder, put on a sanitary pad, and wait to see if you lose more fluid. Put a thick towel between your legs if the flow is heavy. Then call your caregiver according to the instructions you have been given.

Amniotic fluid does not smell like urine, but instead has a faint odor like that of chlorine bleach. **A foul smell, which suggests an infection, should be reported to your caregiver immediately. You should also call immediately if the fluid is stained brown or green.** Stained fluid means that the baby has had a bowel movement, which could indicate fetal distress. If your amniotic fluid is stained with fetal stool, or meconium, your baby will be monitored extra carefully during labor. Immediately after birth, a pediatrician will suction your baby to keep her lower air passages free of the sticky meconium.

CONTRACTIONS   These periodic tightenings of your uterus could be your only sign of labor. You may feel the contractions as cramps or as a squeezing sensation in your groin, in your back, in your thighs, or radiating around from your low back to your groin. To make progress in labor, your contractions must get longer, stronger, and closer together.

How to Tell If You're in Labor

It's not always easy to tell if you are in labor, even if you've given birth before. You may have several hours of contractions one day, convincing you that you're in labor, but then the process simply stops. People call this start-again-stop-again labor **false labor.** It can be very frustrating.

To see if you're in true labor, try these measures:

▲ Walk. True labor typically intensifies when you stay upright and move around.

▲ Change positions or activity. True labor will usually continue no matter what you do, while false labor often goes away when you change positions.

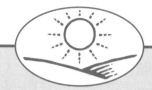

Longer, Stronger, and Closer Together

How long are your contractions?

Time your contractions to see how long each lasts. Early in labor, contractions may be as short as 30 to 40 seconds. As you approach the pushing stage of labor, your contractions may last for 90 to 100 seconds. Depending on how far you live from the hospital or birthing center, your caregiver may ask you to stay home until your contractions are at least 60 seconds long.

How strong are your contractions?

If you can still walk and talk through them, you are probably in very early labor. Your caregiver may suggest that you stay at home, where you can be comfortable, until you can no longer walk or talk through a contraction.

How close together are your contractions?

Time your contractions from the start of one to the start of the next. Many caregivers suggest that women wait to call until their contractions have been five minutes apart for at least one hour and have begun to get closer together. Instructions may be very different if you are already dilated, live far from the hospital, or have a history of rapid labor. Ask your own caregiver for instructions on when to call.

▲ Drink several glasses of water. False labor often occurs as the result of dehydration, so drinking water will stop it. Drinking won't stop real labor, and it's good for you and your baby.

▲ Take a bath or shower. Warm water relaxes you and soothes pain, and standing in the shower can strengthen true labor contractions. To guard against the possibility of infection, some caregivers prefer that you shower instead of bathe if your bag of waters has broken.

▲ Watch your contractions to see if they change. In contrast to real labor contractions, false labor contractions tend to stay the same or get weaker and farther apart—they don't get longer, stronger, and closer together.

▲ Call your caregiver to describe your contractions. If you call when you are about to have a contraction, your caregiver can listen to you try to talk or breathe through one.

Important Calls

Your birth attendant should provide you with instructions about when to call if you think you are in labor. Use these instructions as a guideline, but never hesitate to call if you have questions. Your caregiver may want you to come into the office for an exam or may suggest that you leave for the hospital or birthing center, where you'll be examined.

If a doula will assist you during the birth (see page 151), you may want to call her when you think you are beginning labor. You will also need to contact the people who have agreed to watch any older children. Experienced mothers advise against notifying anyone who hasn't been invited to be present for the birth with the exception of your very closest friends and relatives.

Packing for the Hospital or Birthing Center

A few weeks before your due date, pack a bag for labor that includes some of these items for labor and afterward:

- ▲ lip gloss or petroleum jelly to keep your lips moist;
- ▲ cornstarch or oil for massage;
- ▲ review sheets or childbirth magazines provided by your childbirth teacher (a magazine also makes a good fan);
- ▲ a washcloth to mop your brow or moisten your lips;
- ▲ a watch with a second hand to time contractions;
- ▲ extra pillows (make sure they have distinctive pillowcases so you'll remember to bring them home;
- ▲ eyeglasses so you can see the birth;
- ▲ a snack for your partner;
- ▲ your partner's bathing suit in case he wants to join you in the shower;
- ▲ bottled fruit juice or tea bags, if your hospital does not provide them;
- ▲ a rolling pin or massage roller for back pressure;
- ▲ a picture to use as a focal point for relaxation;

▲ musical tapes or CDs to set the mood, and a tape or CD player;

▲ a toothbrush and toothpaste and, if you like, mouthwash or breath drops;

▲ a brush and comb;

▲ a pair of warm socks, slippers, a robe, and, if you like, a short nightie to wear instead of a hospital gown (since anything you wear in labor is apt to get drenched in various body fluids, bring old clothes);

▲ two nursing bras, if you plan to breastfeed;

▲ a camera and film or a videorecorder and tapes (ask your caregiver's permission if you want to photograph or film the birth);

▲ phone numbers of people to call after the birth, along with a phone card, if you have one;

▲ note cards and stamps to notify friends you can't reach by phone;

▲ a travel clock; and

▲ small change for the newspaper or phone calls.

Before you leave the hospital or birthing center, your partner should bring these things:

▲ an outfit for your baby to wear home, washed to soften it;

▲ a roomy outfit for you (your prepregnancy clothes may not fit for several weeks); and

▲ a car seat to keep your baby safe on her very first car ride (see page 160).

Hospital Admission Procedures

If you've called your caregiver, the hospital staff should be expecting your arrival. Your first exam may be performed in the room where you'll continue your labor or in a separate examining room. If an internal exam confirms that you're in labor, a nurse will give you a hospital gown and request a urine sample. The prep (shaving of pubic hair and enema), which used to be standard procedures (see page 135), is rarely used in most hospitals nowadays. If you haven't had a bowel movement recently, though, you may want to request an enema (see page 135). Stay on the toilet if you can until you've expelled the works, which could take as long as half an hour. Your contractions may feel stronger while you're on the toilet.

The labor nurse will listen to your baby's heart tones and check your blood pressure and temperature. In many hospitals, the baby's heartbeat and the mother's contractions are monitored with an electronic fetal monitor (see page 136) for about half an hour at the beginning of labor and then at regular intervals thereafter. You may have instead made arrangements to have telemetry monitoring or ausculation (see page 137).

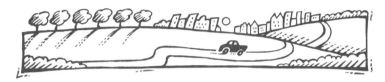

---❤---

Labor: In Stages

The events of labor can be divided into four stages. During the **first stage,** which is the longest, progressively stronger uterine contractions cause your cervix (the necklike bottom portion of the uterus) to thin out and dilate. This stage ends when the cervix, approximately 10 centimeters (4½ inches) dilated, has completely opened around the baby's head. The **second or pushing stage** begins with full dilation of the cervix and ends with the baby's birth. The **third stage** culminates with the delivery of the placenta, or afterbirth. The **fourth stage** begins after the delivery of the placenta and ends one to two hours later when the mother's condition is stable.

Use the next sections as a general guideline to help you go through labor, but keep in mind that your own labor may proceed very differently. Even if you've given birth before, you can't know just what to expect; this labor will be different. To prepare yourself for the unknown, take a childbirth class (see page 123), but always remember to expect the unexpected.

First Stage of Labor

EARLY ACTIVE PHASE, 0 TO 3 CENTIMETERS

The length of this phase varies: One mother's cervix might dilate to 3 centimeters before she even begins labor; another mother may spend several days with uncomfortable contractions before her cervix dilates that far. You can expect mild to moderate contractions, lasting 45 to 60 seconds, at intervals from 20 minutes apart down to about 5 minutes apart. You may feel confident and excited or a bit confused, wondering, "Is this really it?"

Possible symptoms:
- ▲ bloody mucus discharge
- ▲ loose stools
- ▲ nausea
- ▲ chills
- ▲ leaking membranes

What to do:

- ▲ Alternate between activities that relax you (taking a warm bath or shower, getting a massage, listening to music, sleeping, watching television or a movie) and those that may promote the progress of labor, such as walking or nipple stimulation (see page 166).
- ▲ Recheck your packed bag, or, for a home birth, prepare your bed and get out the supplies you'll need.
- ▲ Pack a fresh snack for your labor partner—choose foods whose smells won't bother you—and, if you like, some frozen juice bars for yourself.
- ▲ If you are hungry, eat a low-fat, high-energy snack (toast or crackers with jam or honey, cereal, or soup), and drink plenty of fluids, such as water or diluted juice.
- ▲ Time your contractions to see how long each lasts and how far apart they are.
- ▲ Begin using patterned breathing, if you like, when you can no longer walk or talk during a contraction.
- ▲ Empty your bladder every hour or two.
- ▲ Call your caregiver to report a temperature over 99.5 degrees Fahrenheit, ruptured membranes, or progressing contractions, or to ask questions.

What your doctor or midwife may do:
- ▲ remain available for phone consultation, and,
- ▲ if you have been in nonprogressing labor for many hours and cannot sleep, suggest sleeping medication to allow you to rest and promote active labor.

What your partner(s) can do to help:

- ▲ help you alternate relaxing with stimulating activities,
- ▲ help you stay occupied,
- ▲ time your contractions,
- ▲ offer you food and beverages, and
- ▲ help you get ready to leave for the hospital or birthing center.

ACTIVE PHASE, 4 TO 7 CENTIMETERS

Once you are in active labor, your cervix will dilate, on the average, 1 to 2 centimeters per hour. You can expect moderate to strong contractions, lasting at least a minute and coming closer together than every 5 minutes. Your contractions may be strong enough so that you can't walk or talk through them. As you begin or continue your breathing and relaxation techniques, you may feel the need to concentrate and become impatient with distractions. If labor has gone on for a long time, fatigue can pose a challenge.

Possible symptoms:

- ▲ nausea and vomiting
- ▲ a dry mouth
- ▲ loose stools
- ▲ a flushed, sweaty face
- ▲ back pain between and during contractions
- ▲ a rupturing of the membranes

What to do:

- ▲ Go to the hospital or birthing center after talking to your caregiver. For a home birth, have your caregiver come to the house.
- ▲ Use pillows to relax in a comfortable position.
- ▲ Change positions especially if you have a backache (see "Back Labor," page 176).
- ▲ Between contractions, walk to help labor progress and ease pain.
- ▲ Use breathing, relaxation, and attention-focusing techniques that help you cope.
- ▲ Keep drinking clear fluids.
- ▲ Empty your bladder every hour or two.

Back Labor

About three or four out of ten mothers experience lower back pain that doesn't completely disappear between contractions. The usual cause is that the baby, instead of facing the mother's back, faces forward. In this position, the baby's skull puts painful pressure on the mother's lower back and spine. Until the baby turns around, labor is usually painful and progress slow. To cope, try these tips:

▲ Change positions every half hour or so: Try standing and leaning, the all-fours position, side-lying, sitting up and leaning forward, squatting, kneeling, half-kneeling and half-squatting, or sitting in a rocking chair (see pages 128 to 130).

▲ Get firm pressure on your back from your partner's fist, heel, or from a hard object such as a rolling pin. Or have your partner stand behind you and with his hands, firmly squeeze your hips together.

▲ Ask for hot or cold packs applied to your lower back.

▲ Try a warm shower or bath, with the spray directed at your back.

▲ If you need to lie on your back for a vaginal exam, lie on your fists or a hard object, and switch out of this position as soon as you can.

What your doctor, midwife, or labor nurse may do:
- ▲ check your contractions for their length, strength, and frequency;
- ▲ check your vital signs (blood pressure, pulse, and temperature);
- ▲ check the baby's heart tones;
- ▲ examine you internally to determine your progress;
- ▲ tell you what to expect;
- ▲ rupture your membranes (see "Amniotomy," page 139) to speed labor; and

▲ offer medication, such as narcotics (see page 149) or an epidural (see page 150).

What your partner(s) can do to help:

- ▲ time your contractions;
- ▲ encourage you to drink clear fluids;
- ▲ remind you to urinate every hour or two;
- ▲ help you relax, use patterned breathing, and change into different positions;
- ▲ offer massage, help in the shower, lip balm, warm compresses on your back or thighs, or a cool washcloth on your forehead; and
- ▲ talk about your progress and praise your efforts.

TRANSITION PHASE, 8 TO 10 CENTIMETERS

During this intense part of labor, which typically lasts for 15 to 90 minutes, the cervix dilates very quickly. You can expect very strong, multiple-peak contractions, lasting about 90 seconds and coming about every two to three minutes. These contractions may be accompanied by a strong urge to push. Because pushing too soon could delay progress by swelling the cervix, get checked before pushing. You may feel very sleepy and confused. Many women also get discouraged, panicky, or irritable.

Possible symptoms:

- ▲ increased vaginal discharge
- ▲ shaking of the upper thighs
- ▲ cramps in the legs or buttocks
- ▲ pressure on the vagina or rectum—the feeling of needing to have a bowel movement
- ▲ back pain, because the baby is facing forward or has descended deep into the pelvis
- ▲ nausea, vomiting, belching, or hiccuping
- ▲ cold feet
- ▲ a flushed, sweaty face
- ▲ a possible urge to push
- ▲ a rupturing of the membranes

What to do:

- ▲ Remember that your baby will be born soon.
- ▲ Concentrate on getting through just one contraction at a time.

▲ Use the breathing and relaxation techniques you learned in your childbirth class.

▲ Open your eyes and focus on your partner if you cannot concentrate with your eyes closed.

▲ Pant or blow to control an urge to push until your caregiver or a nurse has checked to be sure you're ready. Have your partner call someone to check you, if necessary.

▲ Change positions for comfort.

▲ Empty your bladder every hour.

What your doctor, midwife, or labor nurse may do:

▲ continue checking your condition and your baby's well-being,

▲ check your cervix if you feel a need to push, and

▲ rupture your membranes if they haven't already broken (see "Amniotomy," page 139).

What your partner(s) can do to help:

▲ be firm and encouraging, and remind you to take one contraction at a time;

▲ call your name to get your attention;

▲ maintain eye contact with you to keep your attention;

▲ demonstrate breathing patterns learned in childbirth classes;

▲ time your contractions;

▲ sponge your face between contractions;

▲ offer you comforts such as ice chips, warm or cool compresses, or a back massage;

▲ remind you to pant or blow if you start to push;

▲ call someone to check you if you begin to push involuntarily;

▲ stay with you; and

▲ keep a thick skin, since you may become angry and hostile (fortunately, this mood is temporary).

Second Stage of Labor

During this stage, you'll work with the contractions, pushing to deliver your baby. For a first baby, this stage usually lasts one to two hours. Later babies are born after an average of about 20 to 30 minutes. It's normal for some mothers to push for only ten minutes, and for others to take several hours.

Now you'll bear down at the peak of each contraction. You can expect moderate to strong contractions every two to five minutes, lasting about a minute each. You may feel exhausted when you begin or after prolonged pushing. But many mothers get a second wind and labor with a sense of growing excitement.

Possible symptoms:

- ▲ a temporary break in the contractions as the second stage begins
- ▲ an increasingly strong urge to push as the baby descends
- ▲ a bloody vaginal discharge
- ▲ an intense pressure and stretching as the baby moves down the vagina
- ▲ a brief burning sensation as the baby's head presses against the perineum (the area between your vagina and anus)

What to do:

- ▲ Relax your neck and throat muscles, your legs, and your bottom.
- ▲ Don't worry if you expel feces while pushing; this is normal.
- ▲ Take a couple of long, slow breaths at the beginning and end of each pushing contraction.
- ▲ Follow your instinct to bear down several times at the peak of each contraction.
- ▲ To avoid a drop in your baby's heartbeat hold your breath for no longer than six or seven seconds with each push. If you can, push with a slow, forceful exhaled breath.
- ▲ Experiment with different positions, such as squatting or side-lying. Squatting takes advantage of gravity, and side-lying promotes comfort (see page 129).

▲ Pant or blow if your caregiver says to stop pushing, to ease out the baby's head gradually.

▲ Open your eyes and watch your baby being born.

What your doctor, midwife, or labor nurse may do:

▲ encourage you to get in a different position, such as a squat, if your progress is slow;

▲ check your baby's heart tones and your blood pressure;

▲ massage your perineum to help it stretch or apply warm compresses to help you relax;

▲ remind you to stop pushing as your baby's head crowns;

▲ offer a mirror so you can see the birth; and

▲ invite you to touch your baby's head or lift out your baby's shoulders.

What your partner(s) can do to help:

▲ encourage your pushing efforts,

▲ support you in the position you prefer,

▲ remind you to relax your perineum and to watch what is happening,

▲ encourage you to breathe slowly a couple of times before and after each push, and

▲ watch the birth.

Third Stage of Labor

During this stage you'll deliver the placenta, or afterbirth. You or your partner may be invited to hold your newborn while you await the birth of the placenta. Contractions will stop after birth, then begin again. As your uterus continues to contract, the placenta peels off the uterine wall.

After your baby's birth you may feel exhausted. You'll probably be relieved that the hard work of birth is over. You may or may not fall immediately in love with your baby. But you will probably be excited and curious about this newest member of your family.

Possible symptoms:

▲ vaginal bleeding

▲ shaking

▲ chills
▲ pain from contractions

What to do:

▲ Focus on your breathing to ease the pain.
▲ Push the placenta out when told to do so.
▲ Hold your baby.
▲ Offer your baby the breast within the first hour or two.
▲ If you like, ask to see the placenta. You may want to have it refrigerated or frozen to bury later.

What your doctor, midwife, or labor nurse may do:

▲ direct you when to push,
▲ check your baby's general condition,
▲ delay the baby's eye treatment (see page 192) until the family has had some time together,
▲ encourage you to hold and feed your baby, and
▲ collect umbilical cord blood (see page 155).

What your partner(s) can do to help:

▲ cut the umbilical cord shortly after birth, unless you prefer to do this yourself;
▲ praise you for your efforts during labor; and
▲ hold the baby or support you as you hold the baby.

Fourth Stage of Labor

After the placenta comes out, your caregiver or nurse will be watching you and your baby closely for an hour or two. Your uterus will continue to contract, and you will begin to experience a bloody vaginal discharge called lochia. You may feel cold, tired, and hungry—or exhilarated and full of energy. You will probably be happily absorbed in exploring your newborn. Later you may want to talk about how labor went and ask how to relieve some common discomforts.

Possible symptoms:

▲ trembling legs
▲ uterine contractions, sometimes called afterpains
▲ perineal swelling or discomfort from stretching or stitches

What to do:

- ▲ Ask for a warm blanket to be placed over you and your baby.
- ▲ Hold and enjoy your baby.
- ▲ Begin breastfeeding.
- ▲ Request an ice pack to decrease perineal swelling.
- ▲ Use breathing and relaxation techniques to cope with afterpains and uterine massage.
- ▲ Ask your caregiver to show you how to massage your own uterus.

What your doctor, midwife, or labor nurse may do:

- ▲ stitch an episiotomy or tear, if necessary;
- ▲ offer you a warm blanket;
- ▲ monitor your blood pressure and bleeding;
- ▲ massage your uterus and teach you to massage it to keep it contracted;
- ▲ apply ice to decrease perineal swelling;
- ▲ help you begin nursing; and
- ▲ help you to the bathroom to urinate.

What your partner(s) can do to help:

- ▲ hold, touch, and admire the baby;
- ▲ offer you comforts such as a cool drink or hot tea, a wet washcloth on your brow, or a meal;
- ▲ review the birth experience with you;
- ▲ go to the hospital nursery if the baby is moved there; and
- ▲ call family and friends to share the news.

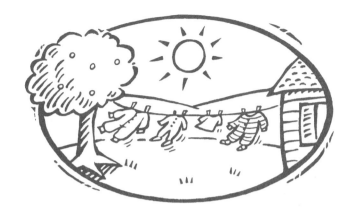

CHAPTER 9

It's a Baby!

After the birth, you face two enormous tasks: recovering from labor and learning to care for your new baby. Fortunately, plenty of friendly help is available in the hospital or birthing center and at home. You simply need to ask for it.

❤ Looking After Yourself

After giving birth in a hospital, you may stay in the same room or be moved to a postpartum room. Your postpartum nurse will show you how to take care of yourself and answer your questions. At home or in a birthing center, a midwife will probably fill the same role.

Helping Your Body Recover

Your body will make many adjustments in the first hours and days after delivery. Some conditions, such as post-delivery vaginal discharge (lochia) and recovery from a cesarean, continue for several weeks. The following sections discuss your body's changes after delivery and suggest steps you can take to make your recovery go more smoothly.

AFTERPAINS   Your uterus must contract after the birth to prevent excessive bleeding and return to its prepregnant size. These contractions, called afterpains, may be painful for a day or two, particularly if you have given birth before, and especially when you breastfeed.

For several hours after the delivery, your nurse or midwife will repeatedly check your uterus and massage it to make sure it stays hard. Or she may show you how to do this.

If you have strong afterpains or the massage hurts, use the childbirth techniques of relaxing, focusing, and breathing that you learned in childbirth class. You may also want to request a mild pain-killer, such as acetaminophen or ibuprofen, or you may need a stronger pain-killer, such as codeine. Less medication will reach your baby if you take a pill just before or just after you nurse.

BATHING   If your hospital postpartum room has a shower, as most do, you can use it as soon as you feel steady on your feet. And you'll want to, because it's normal to sweat heavily after giving birth, as the body rids itself of extra fluids.

Tub bathing has traditionally been forbidden in the early postpartum period to cut the risk of infection. But bathing in a clean tub shouldn't cause a postpartum infection. What's more, a bath may soothe your sore bottom better than a shower. Ask your caregiver about whether you can take tub baths at home.

Since the rapid fluid loss that follows delivery may make you feel faint in the shower or tub, be sure that a nurse or family member stays close by when you bathe.

THE BOTTOM LINE   During delivery, the perineum—the muscular area between the vagina and anus—stretches. This stretching alone will make you feel sore after giving birth. You may also have stitches from a tear or episiotomy, which can cause further pain, swelling, and pulling. For **perineal pain,** caregivers typically advise ice packs for 12 to 24 hours, followed by frequent soaks in a shallow warm sitz bath. Taking a leaf from sports medicine, some experts recommend ice-cold sitz baths beyond the first day if severe swelling and pain persist. Ice numbs pain and reduces swelling, while heat promotes circulation and provides comfort.

In addition, you can ease perineal pain by—

▲ walking and doing frequent Kegels (see page 63) to boost circulation;

▲ using witch hazel compresses after urinating (you can make your own by soaking sanitary napkins in witch hazel—for extra comfort, refrigerate the pads before using them);

▲ doing a Kegel while changing positions;

▲ sitting flat rather than leaning to one side, which pulls on stitches; and

▲ urinating in the shower, to lessen the stinging as urine passes over a tear or stitches.

For two to six weeks after the birth, you'll have a vaginal discharge called **lochia.** Lochia begins with bleeding like a heavy period, then tapers off, gradually fading to pink, then turning brown, yellowish, and white before disappearing. To avoid infection, use sanitary napkins instead of tampons to catch this flow.

Shortly after the birth, you'll be asked to try to urinate. Frequent **urination** allows your uterus to contract more efficiently. Like sweating, peeing also clears your body of the fluids you needed during pregnancy to support an expanded blood volume. If you have trouble urinating, try these tips:

▲ Turn on the tap and run some warm water over your hand, or just listen to the water running.

▲ Ask your nurse for privacy.

▲ Put water in the plastic bottle you'll be given for post-toilet use, and squirt the water on your bottom as you sit on the toilet.

▲ Drink at least eight glasses of water or other fluids each day to keep your urine diluted so that it will burn less when you urinate.

Drinking a lot of fluids also helps prevent **constipation.** Many new mothers hesitate to move their bowels for fear that bearing down will tear their stitches or hurt their hemorrhoids (see page 89). In fact, it's normal not to need to move your bowels for as many as three or four days after delivery. But it will be more comfortable for you to have a bowel movement, when you're ready, if you keep your stools soft. Here's how:

▲ Eat high-fiber foods, such as fresh fruits and vegetables, whole-grain breads and cereals, and prunes or prune juice.

▲ Minimize your use of post-cesarean narcotic painkillers, which are constipating.

▲ Walk.

▲ Don't put off the urge to move your bowels.

If you become constipated ask your caregiver about using a stool softener, glycerin suppository, or enema.

You may have had **hemorrhoids** during pregnancy (see page 89), or they may have made their first appearance as you pushed your baby out. During the postpartum period, hemorrhoids can be itchy and painful. To ease the pain:

▲ Avoid constipation (see page 84).

▲ Use ice packs or witch hazel compresses (see page 185).

▲ Take frequent short soaks in a warm water sitz bath.

▲ After using the toilet, gently replace hemorrhoids in the rectum with your finger.

▲ Lie on your stomach with a pillow under your hips.

▲ Use a lubricating hemorrhoidal ointment (ask for one in the hospital if you need it).

BREAST CARE   All new mothers have yellowish **colostrum,** or pre-milk, in their breasts. Your baby's sucking will stimulate your milk to come in two to five days after the birth. Nursing your baby shortly after birth and frequently thereafter for at least ten minutes on each side helps promote milk production.

When your milk comes in—probably not until after you have left the hospital or birthing center—your nipples may feel sore, and your breasts will probably become engorged: tender, firm, and hot. You can avoid or minimize **sore nipples** by making sure your baby latches on properly (ask for expert assistance the first few times you feed), feeding your baby in different positions, beginning with the less sore side first, and letting your nipples air dry between feedings.

Engorgement typically lasts only a day or two. You may be able to prevent or relieve it by nursing frequently—every one to three hours, day and night, after your milk comes in—until these symptoms subside. The usually recommended treatment—heat in the form of hot showers and compresses—can actually worsen engorgement. In contrast, ice packs used for a short time after nursing may reduce swelling and ease pain. If engorgement causes your nipple to flatten, making it hard for your baby to latch on, hand express just enough milk to soften your areola, the dark area around your nipple. For this purpose, standing briefly in a warm shower may be helpful. Massaging your breast while your baby nurses can also help relieve engorgement and discomfort.

In most hospitals, a nurse or a lactation consultant helps each new mother begin to nurse her baby. At home or in a birthing center, a midwife usually helps with nursing. Ask your helper to show you how to massage your breast and how to hand-express milk. And be sure to ask for the phone numbers of experts to call if you have questions later.

POST-CESAREAN RECOVERY   If you have had a cesarean, you'll need pain relief after your anesthesia wears off. Many hospitals use a long-lasting narcotic injected into the epidural space in the back (see page 145). A few hospitals use TENS (see page 145). Or you may receive narcotics injections, pills, or patient-controlled analgesia (PCA). With PCA, you press a button to add a small, preset dose of narcotics to your intravenous solution whenever you need pain relief. Ask for more medication if you need it. Medication won't hurt your baby, and it can help you care for him and move more easily.

The simplest tasks may seem huge after a cesarean birth. If you have to have a roommate, you may prefer one who has also had a cesarean, because you'll both be moving slowly. If you have a single room, ask whether your partner can stay overnight.

Ask your nurse to show you the best ways to roll over, get out of bed, feed your baby, and walk. For example, to keep your nursing baby off your most tender spot, feed him in the football hold, scooped up in your arm on the side you plan to use for the feeding.

Walking will hasten your healing process. Be sure to ask for help, take it slow, and stand tall when you walk. Walking also relieves the **gas pains** that are a common complaint as the digestive system recuperates from the trauma of surgery. Antibiotics can also generate gas. To minimize it, avoid using a straw and steer clear of hot, cold, or fizzy drinks. Once you start eating regular food, avoid the ones that typically give you gas. In addition, try these tips:

▲ Breathe deeply while holding your hands or a pillow over your incision to ease the pain.

▲ Rock in a rocking chair.

▲ Lie on your back or side with your legs drawn up while you massage your abdomen.

▲ Ask your nurse to insert a rectal tube, a painless procedure that offers fast relief.

You'll need more help at home after having a cesarean. If your partner can't take time off from work, ask a relative or friend to pitch in with housework and cooking for a week or two.

KEGELS AND OTHER EXERCISES   Resume doing Kegels (see page 63) immediately after delivery. This exercise speeds the healing process by promoting circulation to your sore perineum. Begin by doing two or three Kegels an hour, holding each one for a few seconds. Gradually work up to several daily sets of five, holding each for 5, then 10, then 20 seconds. Do a Kegel when you change positions and before doing any abdominal muscle exercise, such as the pelvic tilt.

Your abdominal muscles also require attention after birth. Within an hour of delivery, you can do the **pelvic tilt** exercise, which can improve your posture, strengthen your abdominal muscles, and soothe a sore back. Lying flat in bed with your knees bent, press your waist to the bed for a count of three. Gradually increase to a count of five. After several days, do pelvic tilts in other positions (see pages 65 to 67).

Abdominal muscle separation (see page 65) commonly occurs during pregnancy. If your abdominal muscles have separated, strenuous postpartum abdominal exercise such as sit-ups will only increase the separation and threaten injury to your lower back. On the second or third day after delivery, check your muscles for separation:

▲ Lie on your back with your knees bent, and place your hand flat on your belly with your fingertips at your navel, pointing down.

▲ Raise your head, bringing your chin toward your chest as you breathe out.

▲ As your abdominal muscles tense, they will begin to draw closer together.

▲ See how many fingers fit into the gap between the muscle bands. A gap of one or two fingers is normal after pregnancy, but a gap of three ·or four fingers means you should bring the muscles together before doing other abdominal exercises.

To bring your abdominal muscles back together, follow these steps:

▲ Lie on your back with your knees bent and your hands crossed over your abdomen.

▲ As you exhale, raise your head, while pulling your abdominal muscles toward the middle with your hands.

▲ Hold for a count of five.

▲ Inhale, slowly lowering your head.

▲ Do five to ten repetitions of this exercise at least four times each day. The muscle separation should lessen within a week or ten days.

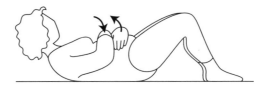

Your caregiver may suggest you wait several weeks before resuming exercise such as swimming or aerobics classes. In the meantime, you can always take walks, with or without your baby. If you have had a cesarean or a complicated delivery, be sure to get specific exercise instructions from your caregiver.

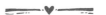

Taking Care of Your Baby

Your birth attendants will have several procedures to complete soon after your baby is born. Your baby will be weighed and measured, and her general healthiness carefully evaluated. But if the delivery has gone smoothly, there should also be ample opportunity for you to hold and care for your new baby yourself.

First Impressions

If your baby is in good condition at birth, she may immediately be placed on your chest, or your caregiver may suggest that you pick her up. You may not even notice that she's just passed her very first test.

THE APGAR TEST   As soon as your baby is born, your doctor, midwife, or nurse will check to see that she's breathing well. Within a minute of birth, and then again when your baby is five minutes

The Apgar Scale

	0	1	2
Appearance (color)	blue	pink body, blue limbs	pink all over
Pulse (heart beat)	absent	less than 100 beats per minute	more than 100 beats per minute
Grimace (a reflex response to suctioning)	no response	grimace	sneezes, coughs, or resists
Activity (muscle tone)	limp	some motion	active motion
Respiration (breathing)	absent	slow or irregular	regular or crying

old, her general well-being is rated according to the Apgar test. In addition to the Apgar rating, your baby will get a quick once-over from your birth attendant or a pediatrician. A more detailed checkup should take place before you go home.

The Apgar scale, named for Virginia Apgar, the anesthesiologist who developed it, rates the baby on five criteria that indicate how well she has come through the birth. Your baby gets 0, 1, or 2 points on each item, for a total possible score of 10. Her initial score predicts what treatment she'll get in the delivery room: whether you can hold the baby immediately or whether she first requires some suctioning, oxygen, a gentle massage, or medication.

Though the Apgar rating doesn't predict long-term health, you may want to know your baby's scores to enter them in her baby book. Typical scores are 8 for the one-minute rating and 9 or 10 for the five-minute rating. A score of seven or higher indicates a baby in good condition.

HOW YOUR BABY LOOKS   As many new parents are surprised to discover, a newborn hardly resembles the adorable, chubby baby of baby-food ads. Don't worry—your baby's looks will improve with time. His head will probably appear too big for the rest of his body, and it may have become temporarily misshapen during birth. His breasts and genitals may be temporarily swollen, thanks to a surge of maternal estrogen. Estrogen also accounts for the milk that may come out of the baby's nipples and the menstrual-like bleeding that appears on some baby girls' diapers. Your newborn's mottled skin may be covered with a cheesy coating of **vernix,** which kept him from becoming wrinkled before birth and which now protects his skin from dry air. Shortly after birth, especially if he arrived after his due date, your baby's skin may appear dry and even peel a bit. This is normal and temporary. So is a deep-red skin color that light-skinned babies may temporarily display as their bodies adjust to breathing. Babies of dark-skinned parents usually look lighter than their parents at birth; their skin hues eventually darken.

You may notice tiny white or yellow pimples called **milia** on your newborn's forehead, cheeks, nose, or chin. The result of clogged sweat glands, milia require no treatment and usually disappear within about a month or two.

Although most babies quickly lose 5 to 10 percent of their birth weight, your baby should regain that lost weight within about ten days. After that, you can expect him to gain about 4 to 6 ounces a week.

In the first few days, many healthy babies display a yellowish cast to the skin or the whites of the eyes. This **physiologic jaundice** results from the breakdown of red blood cells that the baby no longer needs. The byproduct of this breakdown, bilirubin, is typically processed by the liver and then excreted. But because a newborn's liver is immature, unprocessed bilirubin can accumulate and show up in the skin.

Jaundice usually disappears on its own within a few days, if feedings are frequent, since feedings promote bowel movements. Light on the baby's skin also breaks down bilirubin. But because excessive levels of bilirubin can result in brain damage, blood tests may be recommended to make certain that the baby's bilirubin level is declining. If it isn't, the baby will probably be treated with special lights placed over him or wrapped around him in a fiber-optic blanket until his bilirubin goes down, which will probably happen in a day or two.

OTHER POSTNATAL PROCEDURES   The following procedures may be done immediately after birth, or delayed for an hour or so to give you time to enjoy your newborn at her most wide awake and alert. Your nurse or midwife will weigh and measure your baby, noting her length and head circumference, then take impressions of the baby's feet and place identification bracelets around her ankle and wrist (you'll get a matching bracelet). Next, your baby will be dried, diapered, and swaddled, and a cap will be placed on her head for warmth. Soon after delivery, most babies' eyes are treated with silver nitrate drops or a less irritating antibiotic ointment (erythromycin) to prevent eye infections that could be caused by exposure to chlamydia or gonorrhea at birth. Your baby will also get her very first shot—vitamin K—to promote blood clotting.

Care and Feeding

You will have made your decision to breastfeed or bottle feed earlier. Now you will begin the actual task, with help and advice from your nurse, midwife, or doctor. These same caregivers can guide you in learning about other aspects of baby care described in the following sections—though hands-on experience will almost always be your best teacher.

FIRST BREASTFEEDING   For the first hour or two after birth, most newborns are bright-eyed and alert. If you're planning to nurse, ask for help to begin during this wakeful period, when your efforts are most likely to be successful. You needn't rush to breastfeed immediately, but within the first hour your baby will probably begin rooting for the breast, turning his head and making sucking motions. Then you can position him so his face is right in front of your nipple, and pull him onto the breast when he opens his mouth wide.

Early nursing is good for you as well as for your baby. The baby's sucking causes your uterus to contract, minimizing post-partum bleeding. The yellowish colostrum that precedes breast milk fortifies your baby with infection-fighting white blood cells and antibodies. Colostrum also works as a laxative, prompting your baby to eliminate meconium, the fetal stool that contains jaundice-causing bilirubin. Not all babies catch on immediately, though, so don't worry if your baby seems more interested in crying or looking around. You'll get lots of chances to work on breast-feeding.

BOTTLE FEEDING   If you are bottle feeding, your nurse should provide you with room-temperature formula and help you learn to hold your baby with her head slightly raised. It's important, too, to keep the nipple and the neck of the bottle filled with milk so your baby doesn't gulp air.

Your baby's doctor will advise you which formula to use after you go home. Ask how much formula you should give your baby at a time, how to tell when she has had enough, and when it's time to offer more at each feeding. Formulated to approximate mother's milk, most infant formulas are made of cow's milk or soybeans, and fortified with iron. Ready-to-feed formula, the most convenient kind, also costs the most money. You can economize by mixing powdered formula or concentrated liquid formula with water.

Because bottles and nipples come in a bewildering variety of types, experiment with one or two of each type until you figure out which your baby prefers.

Unless you use bottled water labeled "sterile," you'll need to boil the water you add to concentrated or powdered formula. Boiling for a minute or two kills the bacteria or parasites that may lurk in tap or bottled water. According to the American Academy of Pediatrics, you can use your dishwasher or hot tap water and detergent to clean the baby's feeding utensils as long as your water is chlorinated. But if your family uses unchlorinated water or well water, sterilize the items in boiling water for at least five minutes or heat the filled bottles in a pan of simmering water for 25 minutes.

NEWBORN ROUTINES   After an alert period lasting for an hour or two, your baby will probably sleep through most of the next day or two. His rest will be interrupted by several medical procedures, however. He'll receive a thorough medical examination from the doctor you've chosen for him (see page 158) or from a hospital pediatrician. The baby will also have his heel pricked to draw blood to screen for several diseases. All states require testing for phenylketonuria (PKU) and hypothyroidism. Untreated, these rare conditions can cause severe retardation. Depending on which state you live in, your baby may also be tested for galactosemia, sickle cell disease, and several other conditions.

Your doctor or nurse may check the baby's hearing by watching to see how he responds to soft sounds. He may also receive the first of three recommended hepatitis B vaccinations (see page 110). If your baby is a boy, you may choose to have him circumcised (see page 157).

LEARNING BABY-CARE TASKS   Your brief hospital stay gives you a chance to learn to care for and feed your baby under expert supervision. Most new parents feel clumsy and inept at the start. But your baby doesn't know you've never done this before. Remember to be patient with yourself, your partner, and your newborn. You're all just learning your new roles, and you'll have plenty of time to keep learning after you go home. In no time at all you'll feel like a pro.

The hospital staff should volunteer plenty of help. Ask for any additional help you need. Some skills, like breastfeeding, you'll have to learn by doing, but an expert assistant should be standing by during your first few efforts or whenever you ask. If you like, ask your nurse or midwife to demonstrate bathing, swaddling, burping positions, or diapering.

Try to sleep whenever your baby does. If you find yourself awake in the middle of the night, use the time to enjoy your baby or get some extra help from your nurse.

ROOMING-IN   Today most hospitals with maternity services let mothers care for their babies in their rooms, at least during the day. Many hospitals provide 24-hour "rooming-in" for mothers who want it. And some hospitals have eliminated their central nurseries, so that all new mothers room in with their babies.

Keeping the baby in your room gives you a great chance to learn to take care of her under expert supervision. The more time you spend with your newborn, the more confident you'll feel when you take her home.

Rooming-in can be especially helpful in acquainting you with your baby's hunger cues. Most babies sleep a lot during the first 24 hours after birth. Signs indicating that your baby wants to eat include hand-to-mouth motions, head turning, and cooing sounds. If your baby is in your room with you, you won't miss any of these cues, and if you're nursing you can stimulate your milk production and prevent or relieve engorgement by feeding her whenever she awakens. Indeed, one study found that infants kept in their mother's rooms during more than 60 percent of a hospital stay were much more likely to be breastfeeding at one and four months of age than were infants who roomed in less.

Your hospital, however, may not offer 24-hour rooming-in. Even if it does, you may not feel up to taking care of your baby immediately after giving birth. And so you may decide to send your baby to the nursery for brief periods or for a night. In this case, if you are breastfeeding, ask that your baby be given no bottles of sugar water or formula, which can interfere with breastfeeding. Ask, too, that your baby be brought to you whenever she wakens. Frequent feedings will not only boost your milk supply, but they will also give the nurses an important chance to teach you about nursing.

━━ ♥ ━━

Homecoming

The day you bring your baby home will probably be exhilarating and exhausting. Figure out which tasks you must do, which can be done by family members and friends, and which can be skipped. For the first week or so, pretend you're still in the hospital or birthing center. Take frequent naps, and let your family or friends do the housework and cooking so you can take care of the baby and continue your recuperation.

Danger Signs for Mother

Symptom	Possible Problem(s)
Heavy bleeding; lochia that does not decrease with rest, contains large clots, or changes back to bright red after fading	Maternal overactivity; retention of part of placenta
Fever and chills	Infection
Foul-smelling vaginal discharge	Uterine or vaginal infection
Calf pain, redness, warmth, or swelling	Blood clot
Pain or burning while urinating, intense urge to urinate, or inability to urinate	Urinary tract infection
Severe pain in vagina, perineum, or abdomen	Separation of episiotomy or cesarean stitches, or uterine infection
Pain, warmth, or hardness in breast; red streak on breast, or hardness	Breast infection
Chest pain, shortness of breath	Heart attack or blood clot
Headaches, fainting, or vision problems	Preeclampsia (see page 115), which occasionally develops postpartum
Depression, anxiety, or sleeplessness	Postpartum depression

Problems at Home

Your hospital will probably give you a list of numbers to call if you have questions or problems after you go home. Use it, even if your questions seem silly to you. Most hospitals will give you a number, usually for the nursery, to call when questions arise in the middle of the night. Some signs warrant an immediate call to your prenatal caregiver or your baby's doctor.

Danger Signs for Baby

Symptom	Possible Problem(s)
Sleeping more than six hours at a stretch or difficulty waking up to feed	Illness
Nursing fewer than eight times per day	Not eating enough to gain weight
Inconsolable crying	Illness or colic, unexplained crying that usually stops by about three months of age
Fewer than three wet and two dirty diapers a day after the second day; fewer than six wet and two dirty diapers a day by the fifth day	Not eating enough
Breathing problems	Respiratory illness
Vomiting	Digestive infection, allergy, or malformation of digestive tract
Blood in the stool or urine	Illness
Liquid, green, or foul-smelling stools (a breastfed baby's stools are naturally yellow, curdy, and soft)	Digestive disorder or infection
Strong yellow or orange cast to skin or eyes	Jaundice that may require treatment (see page 192)
Fever (armpit temperature over 99 degrees Fahrenheit or rectal temperature over 101 degrees)	Infection or severe dehydration
Anything that seems wrong to you	

INTRODUCING YOUR NEW BABY TO YOUR PET When you come home from the hospital or birthing center, it's best for you to greet your dog while someone else holds the baby. Bring the dog toward the baby gradually, rewarding good behavior and avoiding harsh punishments. Don't leave the dog alone with the baby, and be sure to keep your baby's diaper pail tightly shut.

Introducing a cat to a new baby is much simpler. Simply sit down with your baby and let your cat inspect him. Avoid leaving your cat and your newborn alone; shut the door of the baby's room or install a tight netting over the crib (but remove the netting as soon as the baby can reach it).

SOOTHING YOUR BABY Your newborn may cry a little or a lot. Healthy babies under three months old cry an average of one to four hours a day, increasing their output in the evening and peaking at about six weeks. Experienced parents offer these tips for calming your crybaby:

▲ Feed her.

▲ Swaddle her in a receiving blanket.

▲ Rock her gently in a rocking chair or swing.

▲ Take her for a walk around the block, snuggled against your chest in a cloth infant carrier.

▲ Play some music, or sing.

▲ Hold her against your shoulder.

▲ Lay her on her stomach across your knees and rub her back.

▲ Massage or stroke her tummy.

▲ See if she'll fall asleep to white noise—the sound of the clothes dryer, a fan, or radio static.

▲ Take her for a short ride in the car.

▲ Read a book or the newspaper aloud.

Above all, don't lose your temper. Instead take some slow, deep breaths, and call a friend, family member, or your pediatrician if you need help.

Most babies respond to extra carrying by crying less. But extra carrying may not decrease crying in a baby who has colic. **Colic**— lengthy daily periods of inconsolable crying beginning before one month of age—has long baffled parents, doctors, and researchers. The good news is that colic almost always disappears by six months and that colicky babies usually thrive despite their tears.

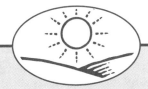

Myths and Facts About Infant Feeding

MYTH: Beer is good for nursing.

FACTS: Alcohol decreases your milk and changes its taste. Although an occasional glass of beer or wine won't harm your baby, some experts advise avoiding alcohol altogether while nursing. Brewer's yeast is rich in B vitamins, but you can add it directly to other foods instead of drinking beer.

MYTH: Babies need to drink water when the weather is warm.

FACTS: Water is unnecessary and in large amounts can even be harmful for newborns. Drink the extra water yourself and nurse your baby more often.

MYTH: It's a good idea to give your baby a bottle when you put him to bed.

FACTS: Putting your baby to bed with a bottle of anything containing sugar—formula, breast milk, juice, or sugar water—can cause serious decay to develop soon after his teeth erupt.

MYTH: Giving your baby cereal will make him sleep longer at night.

FACTS: Feeding your baby cereal won't increase sleeping time. But because formula takes longer for babies to digest, a formula-fed baby may sleep longer than a nursing baby.

If your baby has colic, try these measures:

▲ Hold your baby with pressure against her tummy. For example, lay her face down across your lap while rubbing her back.

▲ If you are bottle-feeding, try a different formula.

▲ If you are breastfeeding, try omitting from your diet for several days possible offenders, including dairy products, chocolate, citrus and other strongly acidic fruits, and gassy foods such as beans and cabbage.

THE BABY BLUES   Many new mothers get the blues two or three days after delivery. Symptoms, which may last up to ten days, include crying spells, moodiness, worry about the baby, and anxiety. Hormonal changes probably play a role in the baby blues. So does sleep interruption. To feel better, try these tips:

▲ Seek support from your partner, friends, or other new mothers.

▲ Sleep whenever your baby sleeps.

▲ Keep your baby in a bassinet by your bed or in bed with you so you don't have to get up for middle-of-the-night feedings. Some experts question the safety of an infant sleeping in the parental bed. If your baby sleeps with you, avoid heavy covers that would restrict her movements, soft surfaces like waterbeds, and pillows and quilts that could obstruct her breathing. Be sure, too, that your mattress lies flush against the bed frame.

▲ Let your housework go for a while, or hire someone else to do it.

▲ Use paper plates.

▲ Order nutritious carry-out food.

▲ Eat plenty of high-protein and easy-to-prepare snacks—such as cheese and crackers, nuts, and yogurt—and drink plenty of fluids.

▲ Spend at least a short period outside every day.

▲ Take a walk or see a movie with the baby, or ask your partner or a trusted friend or relative to babysit while you go shopping.

▲ Make a date with your partner to do something fun.

If your blues linger beyond two weeks or if you have more serious symptoms—overwhelming fatigue despite napping, constant crying, frightening thoughts about your baby, anxiety, or inability to eat or sleep—call your prenatal caregiver. Some of these symptoms may be caused by a treatable thyroid problem or by iron-deficiency anemia. Or you may have postpartum depression, which affects about one new mother in ten. Counseling, medication, or both, are typically used to treat postpartum depression (see "Resources").

Sex and Other Postpartum Issues

There is no specific schedule for when you and your partner should resume lovemaking after you have your baby. Couples' experiences differ in this area. It is important, though, not to rush. And the same is true for weight loss, another matter that may concern you. Your postpartum checkup is a good time to ask questions about these and other concerns.

 IS THERE SEX AFTER BIRTH?   For several weeks, fatigue, soreness, and a crying baby may put sex at the bottom of your priorities list. In the meantime, you and your partner can always hug, kiss, and talk honestly about what—besides a full-night's sleep—might give each of you pleasure.

Eventually you and your partner will want to make love again, and that time may come sooner rather than later. Although the standard medical advice has always been to wait to have intercourse until after the postpartum exam (see page 205), sex can safely be initiated once any stitches have healed, your vaginal discharge has faded, and you both feel up to it. In fact, the muscular contractions that accompany orgasm, similar to Kegel contractions, aid vaginal healing. In addition, if you have sexual problems, you'll be more likely to discuss them with your caregiver at your postpartum visit than you will be to discuss such matters over the phone after you go home.

Women with a lot of stitches and those for whom the mere thought of sex seems overwhelming shouldn't have sex until they feel ready. But if you still feel unenthusiastic about sex several weeks after the birth, you should probably discuss it with your caregiver.

The main thing to keep in mind when you make love after giving birth is this: It gets better. The first few occasions may be painful because of sensitivity from your stitches or sore nipples. Too, the estrogen reduction that follows birth and continues throughout nursing decreases vaginal wetness.

Pain may not pose the only challenge. Your nipples may leak or spurt milk during arousal, a normal response to oxytocin release. Because of their frequent use to feed the baby, your nipples may temporarily be less sensitive and therefore less erogenous, at least for you. Or they may be more sensitive, due to tenderness. You may leak urine during arousal until your vaginal muscle tone returns. If so, report this to your caregiver; it could indicate a problem with healing.

To minimize your discomfort and maximize your fun, try these tips:

▲ Feed the baby first to offer yourselves a better chance to enjoy each other without interruption.

▲ Don't rush into penetration: Start with some music, a glass of wine, a warm bath, or a massage.

▲ Experiment with positions—for example, get on top or have your partner enter from the back—to minimize pressure on your sensitive breasts and perineum.

▲ Use a water-soluble lubricant, such as K-Y jelly, to provide vaginal lubrication.

▲ If you're bothered by milk leaking or spurting, cover your breasts or keep a towel handy, but don't worry about lost milk—your body will keep making more.

▲ Your nipples can offer your partner enjoyment even if this stimulation doesn't excite you now. But tell your partner to lay off your nipples if they are sore.

▲ In general, do whatever pleases both of you, don't do anything that hurts, and question your caregiver about concerns.

▲ Use contraception if you're not ready for another pregnancy (see "Family Planning," below).

▲ Don't forget to do those Kegels (see page 63).

You may be afraid of getting pregnant again, or you may believe you can't get pregnant now. In fact, breastfeeding offers some protection against conception. But you can't rely on nursing to prevent pregnancy unless you're willing to nurse your baby more often and more exclusively than most American women do (see page 204).

FAMILY PLANNING   Right now, another pregnancy is probably the last thing you want. Your top priorities are likely to be getting a full night's sleep and enjoying the baby you already have. That's good, because waiting at least one year before getting pregnant again will lessen your risk of preterm labor. While you're breastfeeding, your periods will probably be suppressed for several months, but they may return as early as six weeks after the birth.

Mothers who bottle-feed usually resume menstruation within about eight weeks. Should you ovulate before menstruation begins again, you could get pregnant without even having a postpartum period.

What method will you use to space your children? Family planning methods vary widely in terms of their effectiveness, ease, and acceptability. Discuss the pros and cons of each method with your caregiver at your postpartum exam. Prior to a postpartum exam, caregivers typically recommend using **condoms** for contraception, because they don't need to be fitted. For extra lubrication and insurance against pregnancy, you could add a spermicide, such as a contraceptive gel, cream, or foam.

Like condoms, **diaphragms** contain no hormones, so they won't interfere with breastfeeding. Your postpartum exam would be a good time to be measured for a diaphragm—or re-measured, since your old diaphragm probably won't fit after you give birth. The **cervical cap,** similar to a diaphragm, may be hard to fit after birth, due to changes in the cervix.

The **IUD** has the advantage of remaining in place for months or even years. One type, the Progestasert, which releases the hormone progestin, must be changed annually. The Paragard can remain in place for up to 12 years. After childbirth, the temporarily thinner uterine wall is more subject to perforation. For this reason, many caregivers prefer to wait several months after delivery before inserting an IUD. IUDs can also increase the risk of pelvic infection, a particular concern for women with multiple or non-monogamous partners. But you face minimal risk for a pelvic infection if you enjoy a monogamous relationship and have no history of sexually transmitted disease. For couples who want effective but reversible long-term contraception, the IUD offers an excellent alternative to sterilization.

Other options for long-term infertility include the **Norplant** implant, a device that releases progestin over a period of five years, or **Depo-Provera** injections, which must be given four times a year. Both of these contraceptive methods are compatible with breastfeeding. Either might make a good choice if you want effective contraception and are comfortable with the idea of taking hormones but cannot tolerate birth control pills for a medical reason such as estrogen-related migraine headaches. Possible side effects include weight gain and irregular menstrual cycles.

Some **birth control pills** are compatible with breastfeeding. Most caregivers advise nursing mothers against standard combination (estrogen-progestin) pills, because estrogen can reduce the milk supply. But many nursing mothers use the progestin-only pill, or "mini pill," because progestin does not inhibit breast milk production. Although progestin passes into breast milk, it poses no risk to the baby, who does not absorb the hormone.

If you and your partner opt not to have any more children, you may choose sterilization. You can get a **tubal ligation** immediately after a vaginal delivery or during a cesarean delivery, or two to three months later as outpatient laparoscopic surgery. Tubal ligation can be performed through a tiny cut just beneath the navel after the uterus has resumed its original position. Some women like the convenience of undergoing tubal ligation when they are already in the hospital to give birth. If a tubal ligation is performed during a cesarean, no separate anesthetic or surgical incision is required. But some couples who think during the stress of pregnancy that they will never want more children later change their minds. In fact, couples who undergo immediate postpartum sterilization are much likelier to regret their decision than those who wait for several months after the birth. So most doctors discourage postpartum tubal ligation right after birth unless a mother is absolutely certain she wants no more pregnancies or has a medical condition that would make a future pregnancy dangerous.

Male **vasectomy** is a much simpler and safer procedure than tubal ligation. This minor surgery takes just 20 minutes under a local anesthetic.

You should consider sterilization by tubal ligation or vasectomy as permanent. Surgical procedures to reverse sterilization are expensive, unreliable, and rarely covered by insurance.

Couples who prefer natural birth control often use the **rhythm** or **fertility-awareness method.** But because it requires taking your temperature each morning after six hours of uninterrupted sleep, this method will probably be impossible to use for those first few sleep-deprived months. Besides, your cycles will probably be irregular, and ovulation unpredictable, for several months.

Although American women are typically warned not to count on breastfeeding for contraception, the World Health Organization endorses nursing as a highly effective natural method of limiting family size for women in less developed countries. In fact, breastfeeding can work here, too. Nursing will suppress ovulation dependably for about six months after birth if you have had no postpartum periods and your baby receives *all* her nourishment and sucking stimulation from you. This means no bottles, no formula, no solid food, no pacifier, and no encouraging the baby to sleep through the night. She should go no longer than six hours between nighttime feedings. For some women, breastfeeding and the resulting suppression of ovulation can also reduce sex drive temporarily.

POSTPARTUM CHECKUP   If you've given birth vaginally, make an appointment to see your caregiver about four to six weeks after the birth. If you have had a cesarean, you'll probably have your incision checked after about three weeks.

At your postpartum appointment—

▲ your caregiver should make sure that your uterus has returned to its original size and position and that any cut or tear has healed;

▲ you will probably receive a cervical exam, Pap smear, and breast exam;

▲ you can discuss your family planning preferences (see "Family Planning," page 202) and perhaps be fitted for a diaphragm, have an IUD inserted, or get a prescription for birth control pills;

▲ you should ask any questions on nutrition, weight loss, exercise, or any other health matters that concern you. List your questions beforehand.

WEIGHT LOSS You can expect to lose about ten pounds—the combined weight of the baby, the placenta, and the amniotic fluid—during the birth, and several more pounds within another week or two. But it takes most mothers at least another month or two, and sometimes longer, to lose the rest of the weight it took nine months to gain.

In your effort to fit into your prepregnancy clothes, keep these points in mind:

▲ Crash diets are a bad idea. Whether or not you breastfeed, you need to keep eating nutritiously to recuperate after giving birth and to care for your newborn.

▲ You should keep taking your prenatal vitamins and iron unless your caregiver advises otherwise.

▲ Since dehydration can fool you into thinking you're hungry, you should drink at least 8 cups of caffeine-free beverages each day if you are formula-feeding and 10 to 12 cups if you're nursing. Drink whenever you feel thirsty, and keep a glass of water at hand whenever you sit down to nurse.

▲ Breastfeeding requires about 1,000 calories a day; half of these calories should come from nutritious additions to your prepregnancy diet. This leaves about 500 calories a day to be drawn from the fat stores you laid down during pregnancy. Since one pound equals 3,500 calories, nursing mothers can expect to lose, on the average, about a pound per week.

▲ Exercise not only perks up your mood, it also burns calories and can tone overstretched muscles. With your baby in tow, walk for 30 minutes each day. Ask your caregiver when you can begin a more structured exercise program.

▲ Contrary to some reports, exercise doesn't make breast milk taste bad, provided a mother drinks enough water before, during, and after exercising. Since some babies object to the salty taste of sweat, however, you may want to rinse your breasts before feeding.

▲ Some nursing mothers lose their extra weight within a month or two; others find that several excess pounds hang on until after the baby begins to eat solid food or stops nursing.

---·♥·---

A Final Word

 You've heard this wistful message before, perhaps from your own mother: Babies grow up with lightning speed. It's true. So stop worrying about doing a perfect job, have confidence in your instincts, and relax enough to enjoy your wonderful new baby!

Further Reading

BABY CARE
Your Baby and Child from Birth to Age Five. Third edition, by Penelope Leach (Knopf, 1997)

25 Things Every New Mother Should Know, by Martha Sears with William Sears (Harvard Common Press, 1995)

The Baby Book: Everything You Need to Know About Your Baby—From Birth to Age Two, by William Sears and Martha Sears (Little, Brown and Co., 1993)

Crying Baby, Sleepless Nights: Why Your Baby Is Crying and What You Can Do About It, by Sandy Jones (Harvard Common Press, 1992)

BABY NAMING
A World of Baby Names, by Teresa Norman (Berkley Publishing, 1996)

BIRTH PARTNERS
Mothering the Mother: How a Doula Can Help You Have a Shorter, Easier, and Healthier Birth, by Marshall H. Klaus, John H. Kennell, and Phyllis H. Klaus (Addison-Wesley, 1993)

The Birth Partner: Everything You Need to Know to Help a Woman Through Childbirth, by Penny Simkin (Harvard Common Press, 1989)

BREASTFEEDING
Nursing Mother, Working Mother: The Essential Guide for Breastfeeding and Staying Close to Your Baby After You Return to Work, by Gale Pryor (Harvard Common Press, 1997)

The Nursing Mother's Companion. Third revised edition, by Kathleen Huggins (Harvard Common Press, 1995)

The Nursing Mother's Guide to Weaning, by Kathleen Huggins and Linda Ziedrich (Harvard Common Press, 1994)

Nursing Your Baby. Revised edition, by Karen Pryor and Gale Pryor (Pocket Books, 1991)

COPING WITH PREGNANCY DISCOMFORTS
The Pregnant Woman's Comfort Guide, by Sherry L. M. Jiminez (Avery Publishing Group, 1992)

EXERCISE
Maternal Fitness: Preparing for a Healthy Pregnancy, an Easier Labor, and a Quick Recovery, by Julie Tupler with Andrea Thompson (Simon and Schuster, 1996)

Essential Exercises for the Childbearing Year. Fourth revised edition, by Elizabeth Noble (New Life Images, 1995)

FETAL DEVELOPMENT
A Child Is Born, by Lennart Nilsson (Delacorte Press, 1990)

HIGH-RISK PREGNANCY
When Pregnancy Isn't Perfect: A Layperson's Guide to Complications in Pregnancy. Third edition, by Laurie Rich (Larata Press, 1996)

LABOR AND DELIVERY
Easing Labor Pain: The Complete Guide to a More Comfortable and Rewarding Birth. Revised edition, by Adrienne B. Lieberman (Harvard Common Press, 1992)

Active Birth: The New Approach to Giving Birth Naturally. Revised edition, by Janet Balaskas (Harvard Common Press, 1992)

NUTRITION
Nutrition for a Healthy Pregnancy, by Elizabeth Somer (Henry Holt, 1995)

POSTPARTUM
Mothering the New Mother: Women's Feelings and Needs After Childbirth. Second edition, by Sally Placksin (Newmarket Press, 2000)

The Year After Childbirth: Enjoying Your Body, Your Relationships, and Yourself in Your Baby's First Year, by Sheila Kitzinger (Simon & Schuster, 1996)

("Further Reading" continued)

You and Your Newborn Baby: A Guide to the First Months After Birth, by Linda Todd (Harvard Common Press, 1993)

PREGNANCY AND BIRTH
The Pregnancy Book: A Month by Month Guide, by William Sears and Martha Sears with Linda Hughey Holt (Little, Brown and Co., 1997)

The Complete Book of Pregnancy and Childbirth. New edition, by Sheila Kitzinger (Knopf, 1996)

A Good Birth, A Safe Birth: Choosing and Having the Childbirth Experience You Want. Third revised edition, by Diana Korte and Roberta M. Scaer (Harvard Common Press, 1992)

Pregnancy, Childbirth and the Newborn: The Complete Guide. Third edition, by Penny Simkin, Janet Whalley, and Ann Keppler (Meadowbrook Press, 1991)

PREGNANCY LOSS
Surviving Pregnancy Loss: A Complete Sourcebook for Women and Their Families. Revised and updated edition, by Rochelle Friedman and Bonnie Gradstein (Carol Publishing Group, 1996)

PRENATAL TESTING
Before Birth: Prenatal Testing for Genetic Disease, by Elena O. Nightingale and Melissa Goodman (Harvard University Press, 1990)

TWINS AND OTHER MULTIPLES
Twins! Pregnancy, Birth and the First Year of Life, by Connie Agnew, Alan Klein, and Jill Alison Ganon (HarperCollins, 1997)

Having Twins. Second edition, by Elizabeth Noble (Houghton Mifflin, 1991)

VBAC
The VBAC Companion: The Expectant Mother's Guide to Vaginal Birth After Cesarean, by Diana Korte (Harvard Common Press, 1998)

Resources

BIRTHING CENTERS
National Association of Childbearing Centers
3123 Gottschall Road
Perkiomenville, Pennsylvania 18074
215-234-8068, www.BirthCenters.org
information on birth and birthing centers

BREASTFEEDING
International Lactation Consultants Association
4101 Lake Boone Trail, Suite 201
Raleigh, North Carolina 27607
919-787-5181, www.ilca.org
referrals to local lactation consultants

La Leche League International
P.O. Box 1479
1400 N. Meacham Road
Schaumburg, Illinois 60173
800-525-3243, 847-519-7730,
   www.lalecheleague.org
breastfeeding information; referrals to local support groups

CESAREAN BIRTH AND PREVENTION
C/SEC
22 Forest Road
Framingham, Massachusetts 01701
508-877-8266
information on cesarean birth, cesarean prevention, and VBAC; list of local support groups

CHILDBIRTH EDUCATION
Association of Labor Assistants and Childbirth Educators
P.O. Box 382724
Cambridge, Massachusetts 02238
617-441-2500
information on and referrals to certified childbirth educators and labor assistants

The Bradley Method
   (formerly American Academy of Husband-Coached Childbirth)
P.O. Box 5224
Sherman Oaks, California 91413
800-423-2397, www.bradleybirth.com
information about Bradley childbirth classes; referrals to certified instructors

International Childbirth Education
   Association (ICEA)
P.O. Box 20048
Minneapolis, Minnesota 55420
612-854-8660, www.icea.org
*information about childbirth education;
   referrals to certified childbirth educators,
   doulas, and postpartum educators*

Lamaze International
1200 Nineteenth Street N.W., Suite 300
Washington, D.C. 20036
800-368-4404, 202-857-1128,
   www.lamaze-childbirth.com
*information about Lamaze childbirth classes
   and parenting*

CHILDCARE AND WORKING PARENTS
National Association for the Education
   of Young Children (NAEYC)
1509 Sixteenth Street N.W.
Washington, D.C. 20036
800-424-2460, 202-232-8777,
   www.naeyc.org
*information on choosing a day-care or
   preschool program*

Families and Work Institute
330 Seventh Avenue, Fourteenth floor
New York, New York 10001
212-465-2044, www.familiesandwork.org
*information on research about families
   and work*

DOULAS
(LABOR AND POSTPARTUM ASSISTANTS)
Association of Labor Assistants
   and Childbirth Educators
P.O. Box 382724
Cambridge, Massachusetts 02238
617-441-2500
*information on and referrals to certified
   childbirth educators and labor assistants*

Doulas of North America
1100 Twenty-third Avenue E.
Seattle, Washington 98112
206-324-5440, www.dona.com
referrals to certified doulas

Natl. Assn. of Postpartum Care Services
194 Parkhurst Boulevard
Buffalo, New York 14223
800-453-6852
referrals to certified postpartum doulas

HIGH-RISK PREGNANCY
Sidelines National Support Network
P.O. Box 1808
Laguna Beach, California 92652
949-497-2265, www.sidelines.org
*network of support groups for women with
   complicated pregnancies*

HIV/AIDS TESTING
National AIDS Hotline
800-342-AIDS (2437)
*information on free, anonymous AIDS
   testing*

HOME AND WORKPLACE SAFETY
National Institute for Occupational Safety
   and Health (NIOSH)
800-356-4674,
   www.cdc.gov/niosh/homepage.html
*information about toxic substances, health
   hazards, and occupational risks such as
   carpal tunnel syndrome*

U.S. Environmental Protection Agency
   (EPA)
800-276-0462,
   www.epa.gov/epahome/index.html
*information on children's health, lead haz-
   ards, safe drinking water, indoor air,
   and other environmental issues*

HOME BIRTH
Association for Childbirth at Home
   International (ACHI)
P.O. Box 430
Glendale, California 91423
323-663-4996,
   e-mail: nbwc@ix.netcom.com
*referrals to birth practitioners, independent
   research on birth*

Midwives Alliance of North America
   (MANA)
4805 Lawrenceville Highway,
   Suite 116–279
Lilburn, Georgia 30047
888-923-6262, www.mana.org
*bibliography on home birth and list of
   members available for referrals*

("Resources" continued)

NAPSAC International
(The International Association of
Parents and Professionals for Safe
Alternatives in Childbirth)
Route 4, Box 646
Marble Hill, Missouri 63764
573-238-2010
*book list and directory on alternative birth
services*

ON-LINE RESOURCES FOR PREGNANCY, BIRTH, AND PARENTING

Ask NOAH About Pregnancy
www.noah.cuny.edu/pregnancy/
pregnancy.html

ATC Parenting Links
http://aboutime.com/links.html

Baby Place
www.babyplace.com

Childbirth.org
www.childbirth.org

Moms Online
www.momsonline.com

Parent Soup
www.parentsoup.com

Parent Guide
www.parentguide.com/bestpicks.html

ParenthoodWeb
www.parenthoodweb.com

ParentsPlace
www.parentsplace.com

ParentTime
www.parenttime.com

PAIN RELIEF IN PREGNANCY AND POSTPARTUM

American Physical Therapy Association
1111 N. Fairfax Street
Alexandria, Virginia 22314
703-684-2782, www.apta.org
referrals to physical therapists

National Certification Commission for
Acupuncture and Oriental Medicine
11 Canal Center Plaza, Suite 300
Alexandria, Virginia 22314
703-548-9004, www.nccaom.org
information on certified acupuncturists

PHYSICIANS AND MIDWIVES

American Academy of Family
Practitioners
11400 Tomahawk Creek Parkway
Leawood, Kansas 66211
800-274-2237, 913-906-6000, www.aafp.org
information about pregnancy and parenting

American Academy of Pediatrics
141 Northwest Point Boulevard
Elk Grove Village, Illinois 60007
847-228-5005, www.aap.org
information about parenting

American College of Obstetricians
and Gynecologists (ACOG)
Resources Center, AP109
P.O. Box 96920
Washington, D.C. 20090
www.acog.org
*send SASE to receive the brochure "Your
Ob-Gyn: Your Partner in Healthcare"*

Midwives Alliance of North America
(MANA)
4805 Lawrenceville Highway,
Suite 116–279
Lilburn, Georgia 30047
888-923-6262, www.mana.org
information on midwives

American College of Nurse-Midwives
818 Connecticut Avenue, Suite 900
Washington, D.C. 20006
202-728-9860, www.acnm.org
information on nurse-midwives

PREGNANCY LOSS

Bereavement Services/RTS
(formerly Resolve Through Sharing)
Gundersen Lutheran Medical Center
1910 South Avenue
La Crosse, Wisconsin 54601
800-362-9567, ext. 4747; 608-791-4747;
www.gundluth.org/bereave;
email: berservs@gundluth.org
*information packet and referrals for
bereaved parents*

Centering Corporation
1531 N. Saddle Creek Road
Omaha, Nebraska 68104
402-553-1200
information for bereaved parents

**PRENATAL AND POSTPARTUM
COUNSELING, AND POSTPARTUM
DEPRESSION**
Depression After Delivery
P.O. Box 278
Belle Mead, New Jersey 08502
800-944-4773,
   www.behavenet.com/dadinc
*information about postpartum depression;
   referrals to local support groups*

Postpartum Assistance for Mothers
P.O. Box 20513
Castro Valley, California 94546
510-727-4610
*prenatal and postpartum phone counseling;
   information on support groups*

Postpartum Support International
927 N. Kellogg Avenue
Santa Barbara, California 93111
805-967-7636,
   www.chss.iup.edu/postpartum
*prenatal and postpartum support;
   referrals to local support groups*

PRENATAL CARE AND BIRTH DEFECTS
March of Dimes
1275 Mamaroneck Avenue
White Plains, New York 10605
888-MODIMES (663-4637), 914-428-7100,
   www.modimes.org
*information on pregnancy, birth,
   and birth defects*

National Center for Environmental Health
Centers for Disease Control and
   Prevention
888 232-6789, www.cdc.gov/nceh
*information on birth defects, such as spina
   bifida, and on lead poisoning*

The Association of Birth Defect Children,
   Inc. (ABDC)
930 Woodcock Road, Suite 225
Orlando, Florida 32803
800-313-2232, 407-245-7035,
   www.birthdefects.org
*information and referrals for parent-to-
   parent support*

SINGLE MOTHERS
National Organization of Single Mothers,
   Inc.
P.O. Box 68
Midland, North Carolina 28107
704-888-5437, www.singlemothers.org
information on single mothering

TREATMENT PROGRAMS
Cocaine addiction
800-262-2463
referrals to local treatment programs

Drug and alcohol addiction
800-662-4357
*printed materials on addiction; counseling;
   referrals to local treatment programs*
800-252-6465
referrals to local treatment programs

Sexually transmitted diseases
800-227-8922
*printed information, phone counseling, and
   referrals to local treatment programs*

Smoking
800-422-6237
printed materials on quitting smoking

TWINS AND OTHER MULTIPLES
Mothers of Supertwins
P.O. Box 951
Brentwood, New York 11717
516-859-1110, www.mostonline.org
support for mothers of triplets or more

National Organization of Mothers of
   Twins Clubs
P.O. Box 438
Thompson Station, Tennessee 37179
877-540-2200, 615-595-0936,
   www.nomotc.org
information and referrals to local chapters

The Triplet Connection
P.O. Box 99571
Stockton, California 95209
209-474-0885, www.tripletconnection.org

Twin Services
P.O. Box 10066
Berkeley, California 94709
510-524-0863
send SASE for publications list

Index